Current Progress in Laparoscopic Surgery

Current Progress in Laparoscopic Surgery

Editor: Dean Griffin

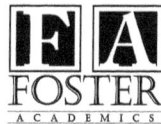

FA FOSTER
ACADEMICS

www.fosteracademics.com

www.fosteracademics.com

FA
FOSTER
A C A D E M I C S

Cataloging-in-Publication Data

Current progress in laparoscopic surgery / edited by Dean Griffin.
    p. cm.
Includes bibliographical references and index.
ISBN 978-1-63242-814-1
1. Laparoscopic surgery. 2. Laparoscopy. 3. Endoscopic surgery. I. Griffin, Dean.
RD33.53 .C87 2019
61705--dc23

Foster Academics,
118-35 Queens Blvd., Suite 400,
Forest Hills, NY 11375, USA

ISBN 978-1-63242-814-1 (Hardback)

Contents

Preface

An operation performed in the pelvis or abdominal region using small incisions with the help of a camera is known as laparoscopy. Laparoscopic surgery is also known as minimally invasive surgery and keyhole surgery. In comparison to the common open surgical procedures, laparoscopic surgeries have more advantages, such as less pain, reduced haemorrhaging, small incisions, lower risk of infections and short recovery time. A laparoscope, scissors, forceps, probes, hooks, dissectors and retractors are some of the common surgical tools used in laparoscopic surgeries. Cholecystectomy, colectomy and nephrectomy are some of the most common laparoscopic procedures. This book includes some of the vital pieces of work being conducted across the world, on various topics related to laparoscopy. The various advancements in laparoscopic surgery are glanced at and their applications as well as ramifications are looked at in detail. This book includes contributions of doctors and experts which will provide innovative insights into this field.

This book is the end result of constructive efforts and intensive research done by experts in this field. The aim of this book is to enlighten the readers with recent information in this area of research. The information provided in this profound book would serve as a valuable reference to students and researchers in this field.

At the end, I would like to thank all the authors for devoting their precious time and providing their valuable contribution to this book. I would also like to express my gratitude to my fellow colleagues who encouraged me throughout the process.

Editor

Ergonomics in Laparoscopic Surgery

Francisco M. Sánchez-Margallo and

Juan A. Sánchez-Margallo

Abstract

Despite the many advantages for patients, laparoscopic surgery entails certain ergonomic inconveniences for surgeons, which may result in decreasing the surgeons' performance and musculoskeletal disorders. In this chapter, the current status of ergonomics in laparoscopy, laparoendoscopic single-site surgery (LESS), and robot-assisted surgery will be reviewed. Ergonomic guidelines for laparoscopic surgical practice and methods for ergonomic assessment in surgery will be described. Results will be based on the scientific literature and our experience. Results showed that the surgeon's posture during laparoscopic surgery is mainly affected by the static body postures, the height of the operating table, the design of the surgical instruments, the position of the main screen, and the use of foot pedals. Ergonomics during the laparoscopic surgical practice is related to the level of experience. Better ergonomic conditions entail an improvement in task performance. Laparoscopic instruments with axial handle lead to a more ergonomic posture for the wrist compared to a ring handle. LESS is physically more demanding than conventional and hybrid approaches, requiring greater level of muscular activity in the back and arm muscles, but better wrist position compared with traditional laparoscopy. Physical and cognitive ergonomics with robotic assistance were significantly less challenging when compared to conventional laparoscopic surgery.

Keywords: Ergonomics, laparoscopic surgery, laparoendoscopic single-site surgery, robotic instrument, electromyography, motion capture

1. Introduction

Despite the many advantages for patients, laparoscopic surgery entails certain ergonomic inconveniences for surgeons, namely, loss of freedom during surgical maneuvers, deriving in an increased incidence of static postures, and adoption and maintenance of forced body postures for long periods of time. Since laparoscopic surgery became more advanced, operating time expanded and, in proportion, so did the levels of mental and physical stress imposed on the surgical team [1]. The combination of these factors with inadequate ergonomic design of surgical instruments may result in decreasing the surgeons' performance and accuracy, as well as the incidence of physical fatigue and musculoskeletal disorders.

The main technical limitations of laparoscopic surgery come from the technical modifications with regard to the open approach. Visual displays are located apart from the surgical field, affecting hand-eye coordination. Furthermore, bidimensional vision causes a confusing loss of depth perception. Specific instruments and fixed access ports limit movements and tactile feedback, worsening surgical performance and demanding greater muscular activity [2]. Design of laparoscopic tools implies a high degree of complexity, requiring manual skills and complementary new knowledge of how to use them. Design of surgical instruments and medical devices, as well as specific location of the monitor, operating table, foot pedals, and other surgical equipment determine to a large extent surgeons' postures while performing surgical procedures and the organization of the surgical team.

The introduction of laparoendoscopic single-site surgery (LESS) has led to a reduction of the number and size of incisions, thus providing aesthetical and emotional improvements to the patients. Positive results have been reported for this surgical approach with regard to postoperative outcomes, recovery time, length of hospital stay, and related costs [3]. LESS inherits the constraints of conventional laparoscopic surgery, adding new technical challenges. Working through a single port implies a defective triangulation, even more lack of coordination, external and internal instrument clashing, forced hands approximation with restrained manipulation, narrowing of the operative field, and possible pneumoperitoneum leakage [4]. Therefore, the use of LESS approach leads to a greater physical and mental workload for the surgeons [5, 6].

Robotic surgery is an increasingly expanding technology that uses human-machine interfaces providing solutions to laparoscopic constraints through enhanced dexterity, maneuverability, stability, and accuracy. Several studies reported lower complication rates and blood loss than conventional laparoscopic surgery [7]. This technology has been also integrated with LESS, and even more complex procedures by means of flexible access devices [8]. The main limitations of robotic surgery are high expenses and maintenance costs, difficulty to use it in low-volume or low-income centers, required experience from the surgical team, and instruments replacement [9].

The term ergonomics can be defined as the scientific study of humans at labor. The main objective of this field is to adapt environments to workers, improving equipment, workplaces, productivity, and training [10]. In this respect, ergonomics applied to laparoscopic surgery is focused on instruments' design and ergonomic assessment, surgeons' posture and workload analysis, surgical environment, and visual displays development [11, 12]. The main objective of this chapter is to review and analyze the ergonomic conditions during laparoscopic surgery and novel minimally invasive surgical approaches such as LESS and robotic surgery, as well as to establish ergonomic guidelines for laparoscopic surgical practice. In order to reach more representative information, studies published after 2010 and with over 20 subjects will be taken into account, excluding the review articles. The content of this chapter will be organized in three main sections: general ergonomic aspects in laparoscopic surgery, methods and technologies for ergonomic assessment in surgery, and ergonomics in minimally invasive surgical approaches.

2. General aspects

In laparoscopic surgery there are some primary ergonomic risk factors for the surgeon such as the body posture, the organization of the work space in the operating room (OR), and the design of the surgical tools.

2.1. Body posture

Laparoscopic surgery has changed the way surgeons interact in the operating field, what is revealed by a change in their posture and movements mainly of the upper limbs. In laparoscopic surgery dexterity is limited due to the fixed access port position, determining the angle of the instruments and instruments motion. Degrees of freedom are restricted from 36 in open surgery to 4 in laparoscopic surgery. This limited range of action leads to surgeons to acquire static, forced, and awkward long-term postures. The primary risk factor for the appearing of musculoskeletal disorders is body deviation from the neutral position. The ideal position for the laparoscopic surgeon is characterized by the arms slightly abducted, retroverted, and rotated inward at the shoulder level; the elbow should be bent at a 90–120° angle; the hands should grasp the instruments with the wrist slightly extended and with the distal interphalangeal joints almost extended, and the metacarpophalangeal and proximal interphalangeal joints flexed at 30–50°; fingers should be abducted and the thumb should be opposed to the index finger [13, 14]. Surgical team and equipment location in relation to the patient also must be considered. Likewise, lower body position can be non-ergonomic, provoking physical stress. Surgeons usually perform long procedures standing with a potential loss of stability and limited possibilities to change their body weight, especially when foot pedals are used [15].

2.2. Working environment

The workplace organization means that every individual member of the surgical team has appropriate space and access to all equipment. A lack of balance between the surgical staff and OR components can lead to work overloads and injuries. The advances in the field of laparoscopy are reflected in the development of optics with higher resolution and improved operational instruments. However, this progress has not always been accompanied by an ergonomic upgrade, which would alleviate some of the problems experienced by laparoscopic surgeons. Besides, some considerations have to be taken into account when using the laparoscopic equipment before and during surgical procedures.

2.2.1. The monitor

The visual information from the surgical scenario is provided by a monitor, which should be adjusted prior to the surgery to avoid undesirable postures for a long period of time. In the horizontal plane, the monitor should be straight ahead of the surgeon and in line with the forearm–instrument motor axis. In the sagittal plain, it should be positioned lower than the surgeon's eye level to avoid neck extension. The most comfortable viewing direction is approximately 15° downward. Viewing distance is highly dependent on monitor size. It should be far enough to avoid extensive accommodation of the eyes and contraction by the extraocular muscles, and close enough to avoid staring and loss of detail [16, 17]. To accomplish precision tasks, the use of an additional monitor near the operative field is recommended, as it improves hand-eye coordination [12, 17].

2.2.2. Operating table

The operating table must be adapted to the surgeon's height and position (standing or sitting). If the operating table is placed too high, muscles apply considerably more contraction force in order to raise and hold the shoulders as well as the elbows. If that position is maintained for a period of time it leads quickly to shoulder muscles fatigue. The table's height should be adjusted in such a way that laparoscopic instrument handles are slightly below the level of the surgeon's elbows. The proper table location keeps shoulders down, and the angle between the lower and upper arm is between 90° and 120° when performing manual work [18, 19]. Lifts can be used in case the table cannot be lowered to a certain height.

2.2.3. Foot pedals

Foot pedals are commonly used during laparoscopic surgery to activate instruments such as electrocauterization, ultrasonic shears, bipolar device, or other tissue welding/dividing instruments. They are often poorly positioned and could demand awkward and unnatural postures. Their main problems are the lack of visual control, unbalanced position of the surgeon, and use of too many pedals during laparoscopic surgery. A possible solution could be replacing them with hand controls when possible. Pedals should be placed near the foot and aligned in the same direction as the instruments, toward the target quadrant and laparoscopic monitor. This allows surgeons to activate the pedal without twisting their body or leg. A pedal with a built-in foot rest is preferable [20].

2.2.4. Surgical instruments

The performance of laparoscopic procedures and the position of surgeon's arms, hands, and fingers are highly dependent on the design of surgical instruments, mainly on the shape of the handle and the tool length. The non-ergonomic designs of handles that are not adapted to the shape and size of the surgeon's hand may lead to discomfort, paresthesias of the digital nerves and muscle fatigue [13]. Surgical instruments should enable surgeons to minimize the wrist flexion and rotation and ulnar deviation, keeping both arms at the sides of their body, and avoiding pressure points on their hands and fingers. Design of instrument handle should be according to the task to be performed, pistol-type handle for tasks that required force and precision-type handle for tasks that require precision [20].

3. Methods for ergonomic assessment

3.1. Body posture

The analysis of the interaction between the surgeon and surgical environment is a determinant factor to evaluate the ergonomic suitability of the working environment and provides crucial information to establish its basic design features. Traditional methods to assess surgeon's postures associated with a specific surgical activity have been based on observation techniques (photogrammetry) by observing the subject directly or using a recorded video [21, 22]. However, assessment methods have evolved and currently it is possible to perform and ergonomic analysis in the OR and using more automated technology. In this section, different methods of ergonomic assessment will be described based on kinematic analysis, muscle activity, or mental stress.

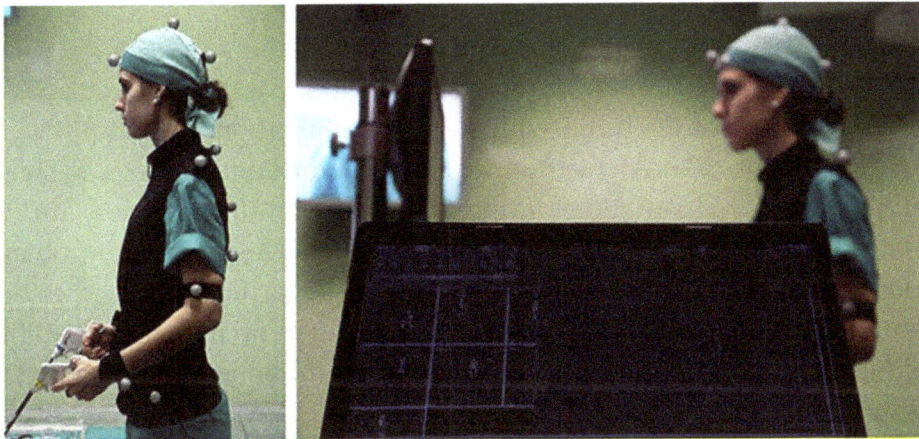

Figure 1. Motion tracking system based on retro-reflective markers. Artificial markers are placed on the targeted segments of the surgeon's body (*left*). A software application computes the kinematics variables during the task execution (*right*).

3.1.1. 3D motion tracking

These measurement systems quantify human movements by means of positional data obtained from artificial markers or sensors placed on the subject's body. Optical tracking techniques are based on color or retro-reflective markers that are identified at the three-dimensional space by a set of cameras [23] around the working space (**Figure 1**). However, these markers may have some occlusion problems in crowded spaces such as the OR, mainly because of the surgical staff and equipment. Another technology for motion tracking is the use of inertial sensors to record in real time the different body segments for subsequent kinematic analysis (**Figure 2**). These inertial measurement units are not affected by visual occlusions, and thus are appropriate for working environments as the OR.

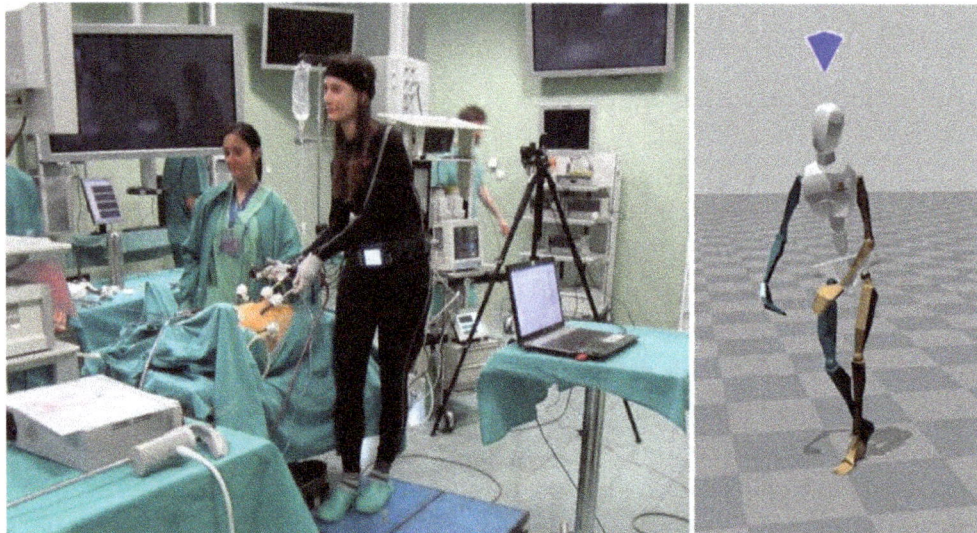

Figure 2. Motion tracking system based on inertial sensors embedded in an elastic suit (*left*). A biomechanical model of the subject is created in real time (*right*).

A set of kinematics variables such as translational and rotational positions, velocities, and accelerations can be computed using the recorded positional data of the subject. Afterwards, the surgeon's posture can be analyzed with standard evaluation techniques such as Rapid Upper Limb Assessment (RULA) method or Ovako Working Analysis System (OWAS). Youssef et al. [24] compared variations in the surgeon's standing position during a virtual reality-simulated laparoscopic cholecystectomy using RULA score. They obtained better ergonomic posture for the between-standing technique, regardless of whether one- or two-handed technique. 3D kinematic analysis was used to differentiate joint variability between conventional laparoscopy and LESS [21], evaluating the influence of the upper body to the head stabilization.

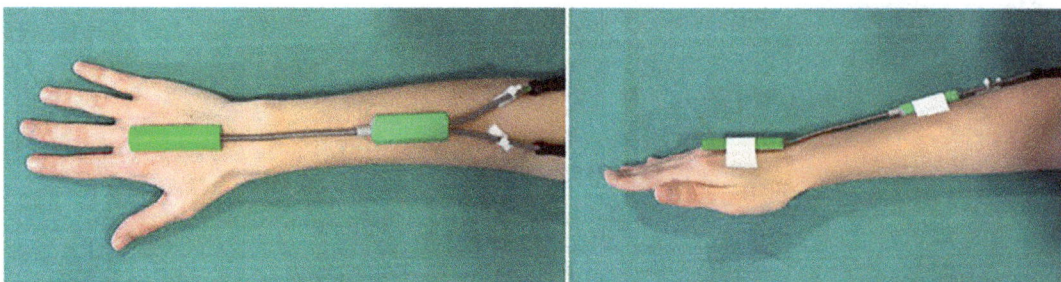

Figure 3. Placement of an electrogoniometer on the hand to record the wrist flexion-extension and radial-ulnar deviation.

3.1.2. Electrogoniometers

Electrogoniometers are devices whose measurement signals (typically electrical voltages) are related directly to flexion-extension or rotation between body segments. These devices should be precalibrated to relate the measured voltage with the angles described by the analyzed joint (**Figure 3**). However, this measurement technology may be difficult to use for certain body segments. Besides, the need to be attached to the body segments and the use of wires for power supply make these devices a cumbersome solution to be used during laparoscopic practice.

3.1.3. Data gloves

Surgical tasks and instruments directly affect the surgeon's wrist and hand position. Data gloves allow for recording movements of the fingers and wrist by means of electromechanical technology or conductive sensors. In the clinical field, these devices have been used in conjunction with virtual reality systems for rehabilitation purposes [25] and surgical planning applications [26]. Recently, this technology has been used to analyze the surgeon's hand movements while using different surgical instruments during laparoscopic practice [5, 8, 11, 27] (**Figure 4**).

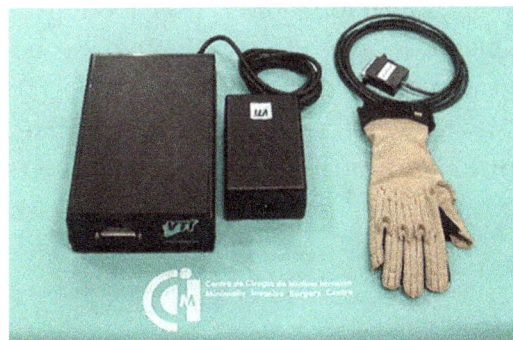

Figure 4. Motion capture data glove CyberGlove® (CyberGlove Systems, San José, CA, USA). This device consists of a series of conductive sensors with resistance flows sensitive to flexion variations.

3.2. Electromyography

Electromyography (EMG) measures the electrical signal associated with the activation of the muscle. This technique allows us to assess the electrical activity of a muscle group during the performance of a task. For data acquisition, electrodes should be placed following standard recommendations, as the surface EMG for noninvasive assessment of muscles (SENIAM) project [28], to ensure the acquisition of EMG signals and reduce potential artifacts.

Several metrics of muscle activity during the execution of a certain task can be computed by analyzing the EMG signal such as the percentage of the maximal voluntary contraction (MVC) [29], the amplitude probability distribution function (APDF) [30], or the muscle fatigue [6]. EMG has been an extended ergonomic assessment method in laparoscopic surgery to analyze the surgeon's postural muscle activity [5, 11], the use of different surgical instruments, and instrument handles [27, 31] (**Figure 5**).

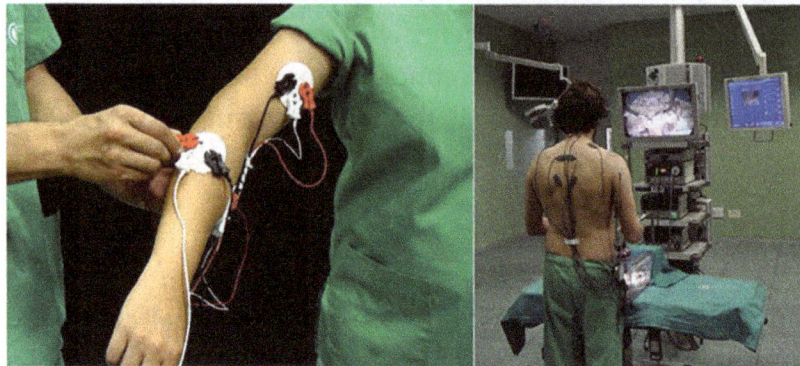

Figure 5. Placement of the EMG electrodes on the right biceps brachii and forearm extensors (*left*). Use of the surface EMG to analyze the muscle activity of the upper body during laparoscopic practice (*right*).

3.3. Force platforms

Force platforms (single or multiple) are used to analyze the body balance during static or dynamic situations. These systems provide information about ground's reaction force against the force exerted by the subject's legs while supporting the body weight. Fan et al. [32] presented an alternative position to conventional flank position in retroperitoneoscopic urological practice. Body balance was assessed during simulated surgical tasks using two separate force plates (Wii Fit balance boards, Nintendo Inc.). They concluded that relative loading between feet was more balanced using the purposed posture.

3.4. Mental workload

Apart from the physical effort, psychological burden of surgeons performing laparoscopic procedures is reported higher in comparison to open surgical techniques [15]. For mental workload assessment, subjective techniques are the most extended methods. The National Aeronautics and Space Administration Task Load Index (NASA-TLX) evaluates six domains: mental demand, physical demand, temporal demand, effort, performance, and frustration during each task execution. A surgery-specific version of the NASA-TLX called SURG-TLX was presented and validated in 2011 [33]. Apart from the physical, mental, and temporal demand, this index assessed the task complexity, the situational stress, and distractions. Studies reported LESS is significantly more demanding than the conventional approach [34]. Training has been proved to improve both task performance and workload in laparoscopic practice [35].

3.5. Questionnaires

Questionnaires are another assessment tool that focuses on gathering information from a population of surgeons. Taking into account studies with at least 100 respondents, a survey to laparoscopic urologists in China concluded that most of them were not aware of the ergonomic guidelines for the OR [36]. Shoulder, neck, back, and hand pain and stiffness were reported as the main physical symptoms during laparoscopic procedures [36, 37]. The surgeon's height, glove size, age, gender, type of instrument, foot pedals, and height of the operating table have been identified as important factors for increasing the musculoskeletal pain symptoms [38–41]. The shape of the laparoscopic instrument handle was identified as the main element that needed to be improved [40].

4. Ergonomics in laparoscopic surgery

A summary of the results from the scientific literature regarding ergonomics in laparoscopic surgery are presented in **Table 1**.

Study	N	Task	Assessment method	Results
[12]	24 novices	Peg transfer with different monitor conditions	NASA-TLX	There are no differences among monitor positions in terms of perceived workload
[16]	20 novices	Suturing on simulator with ergonomic (G1) and normal (G2) settings	Photogrammetry: Neck, shoulder, elbow, and wrist	Optimal ergonomic setting leads to better task performance
[24]	32	Cholecystectomy on virtual simulator with variations in standing position and hand technique	RULA NASA-TLX	Better ergonomic posture for the between-standing technique [30]
[30]	25	Open, laparoscopic, and endovascular procedures	EMG: Back, neck, and shoulder	Open surgery imposes greater physical demand on the neck muscles compared with endovascular and laparoscopic surgeries
[42]	26: 13 with training of the non-dominant upper extremity and 13 without training	Eye-hand coordination task	EMG: Back, shoulder, and forearm	Training the non-dominant upper extremity leads to better alternated use of forearm muscles
[43]	100	Laparoscopic renal procedures with and without foot gel pad	Subjective criteria	The use of foot gel pads improves surgeon comfort and ergonomics during laparoscopy
[44]	28 novices	Nissen fundoplication model	NASA-TLX	Higher mental workload is associated with poorer laparoscopic performance

N: Number of subjects or cases.

Table 1. Reported results for ergonomics in laparoscopic surgery.

In a study with 30 surgeons with different experience in laparoscopic surgery, we analyzed the surgeon's muscle activity in back and forearm muscles during laparoscopic dissection and suturing tasks [29]. Percentage of the MVC of the trapezius, forearm flexors, and forearm extensors muscles was used for assessment of the muscle activity (**Figure 6**). Results showed that the surgeons with a higher degree of laparoscopic experience exhibited a lower level of muscle activity when compared with the novice surgeons. In another study with 50 surgeons, we analyzed the surgeons' hand spatial configuration during the use of two laparoscopic instrument handles, axial and ring-handled [11]. Movements of the surgeon's hand and wrist were recorded by a data glove and the level of wrist disorder was computed by a modified version of the RULA method [27] (**Figure 6**). Results showed that axial-handled needle holder entailed a more ergonomic posture for the wrist joint.

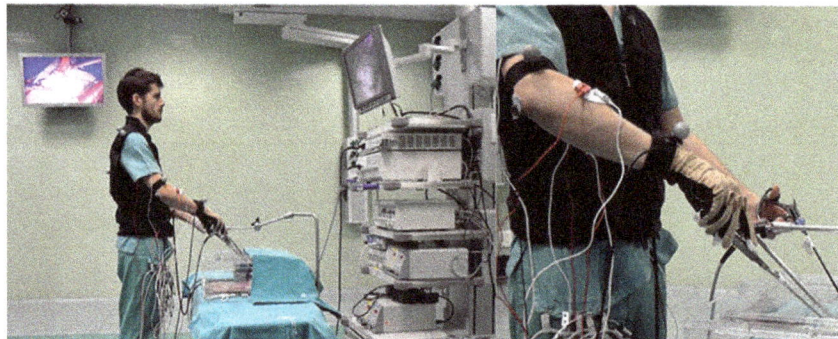

Figure 6. EMG and data glove data acquisition during the performance of laparoscopic tasks on simulator.

5. New surgical approaches

New surgical approaches have been presented to improve surgical outcomes and aesthetics results of patients. However, in some cases these surgical alternatives lead to an increase in technical and ergonomic challenges for surgeons that should be analyzed and identified.

5.1. Laparoendoscopic single-site surgery (LESS)

A summary of the results from the scientific literature for ergonomics in LESS are presented in **Table 2**.

In a study with experienced laparoscopic surgeons we assessed the surgeons' ergonomy during LESS, comparing it with conventional laparoscopic approach [5]. Surgeons performed a dissection tasks on a physical simulator using straight laparoscopic scissors and dissector for the conventional approach, and articulating tip scissors and dissector for the LESS approach (**Figure 7**). Ergonomic assessment was carried out by analyzing the muscular activity, and wrist and hand motion. Results showed that the LESS approach required greater level of muscular activity in the trapezius and forearm extensor muscles, but better wrist position compared with traditional laparoscopy.

Study	N	Task	Assessment method	Results
[34]	48: 25 with LESS and 23 with conventional approach	Cholecystectomy	SURG-TLX	LESS cholecystectomy is more stressful and physically demanding than the conventional approach
[45]	24 premedical college students	Peg-transfer with two articulated and one straight graspers	EMG: Forearms. Electrogoniometers: Wrist. SURG-TLX	The straight instrument requires less muscle activation and wrist deviation
[46]	100 procedures: 50 triportal vs. 50 uniportal	Video-assisted thoracic surgery	Photogrammetry: Head NASA-TLX	Surgeons maintain a more neutral body posture during uniportal VATS, but with greater frustration
[47]	90 patients	Laparoscopic pull-through Soave procedure: conventional, LESS and hybrid approach	Subjective criteria	The conventional and hybrid approach have the same maneuverability and are less challenging than the LESS approach
[48]	175 patients	Different urological procedures	Subjective criteria	The use of conventional laparoscopic instruments is ergonomically feasible and safe in LESS procedures

N: Number of subjects or cases.

Table 2. Reported results for ergonomics in LESS.

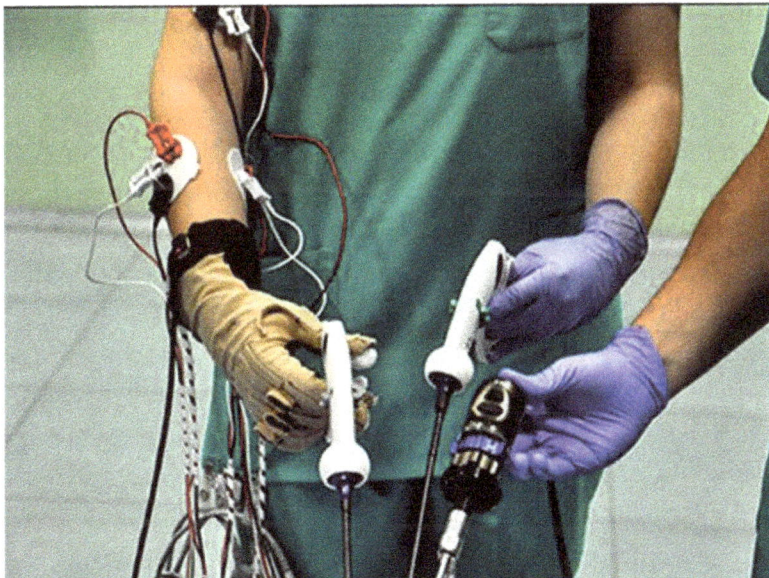

Figure 7. EMG and data glove data acquisition during the performance of hands-on simulator tasks using a LESS approach.

5.2. Robotic surgery

Research has demonstrated the benefits of robotic surgery for the patient such as smaller incisions, reduced blood loss and postoperative pain, and reduced durations of in-patient care. Robotic platforms such as the da Vinci system (Intuitive Surgical Ltd., Sunnyvale, CA, USA) have been presented as a potential solution to the limited ergonomics in laparoscopic surgery.

In a study with surgeons with different levels of experience in robotic surgery, physical and cognitive ergonomic workloads using robotic-assisted and conventional laparoscopy were assessed during the performance of different basic laparoscopic training tasks [49]. Physical workload was assessed by using EMG from back, shoulder, arms, and forearms muscles, and mental workload by means of NASA-TLX index. They concluded that physical and cognitive ergonomics with robotic assistance were significantly less challenging. Another study comparing the use of standard laparoscopy and robotic assistance during intracorporeal suturing on porcine Nissen fundoplication models, medical students reported a lower workload using the robotic assistance [50]. Similarly, Moore et al. [51] reported significantly lower workload and mental effort on the robotic system compared to conventional laparoscopic approach while performing an eye-hand coordination task. Besides, another study using standard laparoscopic tasks during five consecutive training sessions, surgeons (novices and experienced) reported a less frustration score during and after training sessions and higher good mood score using robotic assistance [52]. The Imperial Test Assessment Tool was use to evaluate the frustration level.

6. New surgical devices

In order to overcome some of the ergonomic limitations of laparoscopic surgery, new surgical devices and instrument designs have been developed. In this section, we will review these novel surgical devices presented in the scientific literature. Studies published after 2010 and with no limit of subjects will be taken into account, excluding the review articles.

Several authors presented novel prototypes of ergonomically designed handles for laparoscopic instruments. One example is the Intuitool® laparoscopic instrument (University of Nebraska, Lincoln, NE, USA), which includes an ergonomic handle and a redesigned grasper actuation mechanism in order to create a more comfortable and intuitive handle-tool interface [53]. Büchel et al. [31] also presented a laparoscopic instrument prototype with an ergonomic pistol handle (Volargrip; University Hospital of Trondheim and Surgitech Norway AS, Trondheim, Norway). They compared this tool with two conventional laparoscopic instruments with ring handles. Results showed that each handle except the new prototype caused pressure areas and pain. A pistol grip laparoscopic instrument with a rotatable handle piece was presented by Steinhilber et al. [54]. EMG of the arm and shoulder muscles and wrist's posture by means of a gravimetric posture sensor were used to compare this novel instrument with the use of a conventional laparoscopic handle during the performance of a hand-eye coordination task. Results showed that the novel handle design did not decrease the biomechanical stress of the analyzed muscles, but neutral position of the wrist was more often. Yu et al. [55] compared a prototype laparoscopic grasper with three adjustable handle angles to a conventional instrument during the performance of Fundamentals of Laparoscopic Surgery tasks. Motion tracking and NASA-TLX were used to measure the surgeon's posture and workload. They concluded that the adjustable handle angle laparoscopic tool can reduce ergonomic risks of musculoskeletal strain and allows versatility for tasks alternating between positions.

Another possibility to improve the ergonomics in laparoscopy is by increasing the instrument's degrees of freedom. This is the case of the Radius Surgical System (Tuebingen Scientific Medical GmbH, Tuebingen, Germany), which provides two additional degrees of freedom (deflection and rotation of the tip) and enables the surgeon to manipulate the instrument accurately and precisely in an ergonomic position [56]. This manipulator has been successfully used to treat cases of esophageal achalasia and gastroesophageal reflux disease [57].

Apart from laparoscopic surgical instruments, other support devices have been developed to improve the ergonomic conditions during surgery. This is the case of operating chairs [58] or arm supports [59], whose main objective is to improve the surgeon's ergonomic posture during surgery. A novel portable ergonomic simulator for training of basic laparoscopic skills was also presented by Xiao et al. [60].

6.1. Handheld robotic instruments

New handheld robotic systems have been developed for laparoscopic surgery and single-site surgery to deal with some of their technical and ergonomic limitations. They provide precision-driven and articulating instrument tips, which increase the triangulation, and therefore improve the performance of some surgical maneuvers. One example of these systems is Jaimy® (Endocontrol, Grenoble, France), which provides two additional degrees of freedom controlled by a joystick placed on an ergonomic handle [8]. This handheld robotic instrument was ergonomically compared by means of surgeon's posture and muscular activity analysis with a conventional needle holder during the performance of basic laparoscopic training tasks. Results showed that the use of the robotized needle holder improved the surgeon's posture when compared to the traditional laparoscopic instrument.

The Kymerax™ (Terumo Europe NV, Leuven, Belgium) and DEX™ (Dextérité Surgical, Annecy, France) are other examples of handled robotic instruments for laparoscopic surgery and LESS. We have analyzed the ergonomics of these two surgical devices and compared it to conventional laparoscopic instruments by means of motion tracking, EMG of back, shoulder, and arm muscles, and data glove motion analysis (**Figure 8**). A positive learning curve in performance and ergonomics using the handheld robotic instruments has been reported. There were no differences in surgeon's muscle activity using the robotic and the conventional laparoscopic instruments, except for the biceps muscle. The robotic instruments led to an ergonomically more acceptable posture of the shoulder, elbow, and wrist. We believe that a period of adaptation should be required for this new technology.

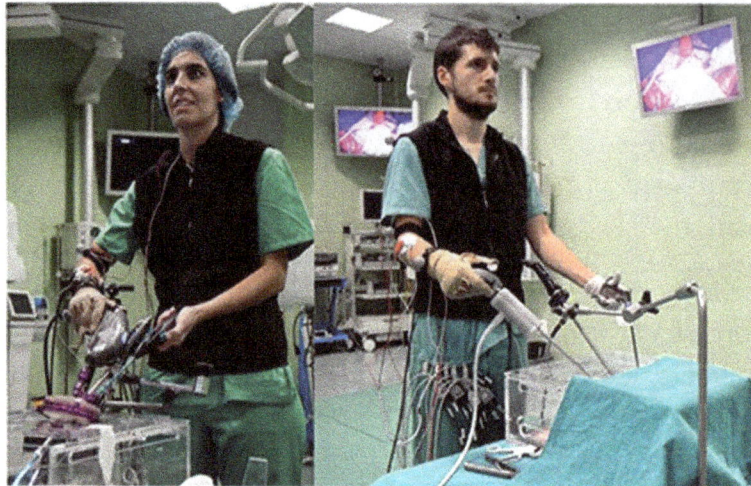

Figure 8. Setup for the ergonomic study in the training environment using (left) the Kymerax™ and (right) the DEX™ handheld robotic instruments.

7. Conclusions

Laparoscopic surgery entails a limited range of movements, which leads to acquire static, forced, and awkward long-term postures. The primary risk factor for the appearing of musculoskeletal disorders is body deviation from the neutral position. The ideal position for the laparoscopic surgeon is characterized by the arms slightly abducted, retroverted, and rotated inward at the shoulder level; the elbow should be bent at a 90–120° angle; the hands should grasp the instruments with the wrist slightly extended. Results from the scientific literature showed that ergonomics during the laparoscopic surgical practice is related to the level of experience. Better ergonomic conditions during surgery lead to an improvement in task performance. Objective ergonomic analysis concluded that laparoscopic instruments with axial handel entail a more ergonomic posture for the wrist joint compared to a ring handle. Regarding ergonomics in LESS, studies reported that this surgical approach is more physically demanding than conventional and hybrid approaches. LESS approach requires greater level of muscular activity in the back and arm muscles, but leads to a better wrist position compared with traditional laparoscopy. Physical and cognitive ergonomics with robotic assistance were significantly less challenging when compared to conventional laparoscopic surgery. Further studies with a greater number of subjects should be done in order to obtain clear evidence-based findings of ergonomics during minimally invasive surgery.

Acknowledgements

This study was supported by the Government of Extremadura, Spain; the European Regional Development Fund (GR15175); and the European Social Fund (PO14034).

Author details

Francisco M. Sánchez-Margallo[1] and Juan A. Sánchez-Margallo[2*]

*Address all correspondence to: juan.sanchez.margallo@gmail.com

1 Jesús Usón Minimally Invasive Surgery Centre, Cáceres, Spain

2 Department of Computer Systems and Telematics Engineering, University of Extremadura, Badajoz, Spain

References

[1] Vereczkel A, Bupp H, Feussner H. Laparoscopic surgery and ergonomics—it's time to think on ourselves as well. Surg Endosc 2003; 17: 1680–2.

[2] Pérez-Duarte FJ, Sánchez-Margallo FM, Díaz-Güemes I, Sánchez-Hurtado MÁ, Lucas-Hernández M, Usón J. Ergonomics in laparoscopic surgery and its importance in surgical training. Cir Esp 2012; 90: 284–91.

[3] Geng L, Sun C, Bai J. Single incision versus conventional laparoscopic cholecystectomy outcomes: a meta-analysis of randomized controlled trials. PLoS One 2013; 8(10): e76530.

[4] Matos-Azevedo AM, Díaz-Güemes I, Pérez-Duarte FJ, Sánchez-Hurtado MÁ, Sánchez-Margallo FM. Comparison of single access devices during cut and suturing tasks on simulator. J Surg Res 2014; 192(2): 356–67.

[5] Pérez-Duarte FJ, Lucas-Hernández M, Matos-Azevedo A, Sánchez-Margallo JA, Díaz-Güemes I, Sánchez-Margallo FM. Objective analysis of surgeons' ergonomy during laparoendoscopic single-site surgery through the use of surface electromyography and a motion capture data glove. Surg Endosc 2014; 28: 1314–20.

[6] Koca D, Yıldız S, Soyupek F, Günyeli İ, Erdemoglu E, Soyupek S, et al. Physical and mental workload in single-incision laparoscopic surgery and conventional laparoscopy. Surg Innov 2015; 22(3): 294–302.

[7] Ficarra V, Novara G, Artibani W, Cestari A, Galfano A, Graefen M, et al. Retropubic, laparoscopic, and robot-assisted radical prostatectomy: a systematic review and cumulative analysis of comparative studies. Eur Urol 2009; 55: 1037–63.

[8] Bensignor T, Morel G, Reversat D, Fuks D, Gayet B. Evaluation of the effect of a laparoscopic robotized needle holder on ergonomics and skills. Surg Endosc 2016; 30: 446–54.

[9] Elhage O, Challacombe B, Shortland A, Dasgupta P. An assessment of the physical impact of complex surgical tasks on surgeon errors and discomfort: a comparison

between robot-assisted, laparoscopic and open approaches. BJU Int 2015; 115(2): 274–81.

[10] Supe AN, Kulkarni GV, Supe PA. Ergonomics in laparoscopic surgery. J Min Access Surg 2010; 6: 31–6.

[11] Sánchez-Margallo FM, Pérez-Duarte FJ, Sánchez-Margallo JA, Lucas-Hernández M, Matos-Azevedo AM, Díaz-Güemes I. Application of a motion capture data glove for hand and wrist ergonomic analysis during laparoscopy. Minim Invasive Ther Allied Technol 2014; 23(6): 350–6.

[12] Rogers ML, Heath WB, Uy CC, Suresh S, Kaber DB. Effect of visual displays and locations on laparoscopic surgical training task. Appl Ergon 2012; 43: 762–7.

[13] Matern U, Waller P. Instruments for minimally invasive surgery. Principles of ergonomic handles. Surg Endosc 2009; 13: 174–82.

[14] Matern U. Ergonomic deficiencies in the operating room: examples from minimally invasive surgery. Work 2009; 32: 1–4.

[15] Gofrit ON, Mikahail AA, Zorn KC, Zagaja GP, Steinberg GD, Shalhav AL. Surgeons' perceptions and injuries during and after urologic laparoscopic surgery. Urology 2008; 71: 404–7.

[16] Xiao DJ, Jakimowicz JJ, Albayrak A, Goossens RHM. Ergonomic factors on task performance in laparoscopic surgery training. Appl Ergonom 2012; 43: 548–53.

[17] Van Det MJ, Meijerink WJHJ, Hoff C, Totté ER, Pierie JPEN. Optimal ergonomics for laparoscopic surgery in minimally invasive surgery suites: a review and guidelines. Surg Endosc 2009; 23: 1279–85.

[18] Berquer R, Smith WD, Davis S. An ergonomic study of the optimum operating table height for laparoscopic surgery. Surg Endosc 2002;16: 416–21.

[19] Van Veelen MA, Kazemier G, Koopman J, Goossens RH, Meijer DW. Assessment of the ergonomically optimal operating surface height for laparoscopic surgery. J Laparoendosc Adv Surg Technol A 2002; 12(1): 47–52.

[20] Berguer R. Ergonomics in laparoscopic surgery. In: Whelan RL, Fleshman JW, Fowler DL, editors. The SAGES Manual of Perioperative Care in Minimally Invasive Surgery. 2005. New York: Springer. pp. 454–64.

[21] Gianikellis K, Sánchez-Margallo FM, Skiadopoulos A, Sánchez-Margallo JA, Aranda JH de M. Head stabilization during minimal invasive surgery tasks: an uncontrolled manifold analysis. Procedia Manuf 2015; 3: 1434–41.

[22] Gianikellis K, Skiadopoulos A, Palma CE, Sanchez-Margallo FM, Carrasco JBP, Sanchez-Margallo JA. A method to assess upper-body postural variability in laparoscopic surgery. 5th IEEE RAS/EMBS International Conference on Biomedical Robotics and Biomechatronics, IEEE; 2014, pp. 76–81.

[23] Lee G, Lee T, Dexter D, Klein R, Park A. Methodological infrastructure in surgical ergonomics: a review of tasks, models, and measurement systems. Surg Innov 2007; 14(3): 153–67.

[24] Youssef Y, Lee G, Godinez C, Sutton E, Klein R V., George IM, et al. Laparoscopic cholecystectomy poses physical injury risk to surgeons: analysis of hand technique and standing position. Surg Endosc 2011; 25: 2168–74.

[25] Jack D, Boian R, Merians AS, Tremaine M, Burdea GC, Adamovich SV, Recce M, Poizner H. Virtual reality-enhanced stroke rehabilitation. IEEE Trans Neural Syst Rehabil Eng 2001; 9(3): 308–18.

[26] Stalfors J, Kling-Petersen T, Rydmark M, Westin T. Haptic palpation of head and neck cancer patients—implication for education and telemedicine. Stud Health Technol Inform 2001; 81: 471–4.

[27] Sánchez-Margallo FM, Sánchez-Margallo JA, Pagador JB, Moyano JL, Moreno J, Usón J. Ergonomic assessment of hand movements in laparoscopic surgery using the CyberGlove. In: Miller K, Nielsen PMF, editors. Comput. Biomech. Med., New York, NY: Springer; 2010, pp. 121–8.

[28] Hermens HJ, Freriks B, Merletti R, Stegeman D, Blok J, Rau G, et al. SENIAM 8: European recommendation for surface electromyography. Enschede: Roessingh Research and Development. 1999.

[29] Pérez-Duarte FJ, Sánchez-Margallo FM, Martín-Portugués I, Sánchez-Hurtado MA, Lucas-Hernández M, Sánchez-Margallo JA, et al. Ergonomic analysis of muscle activity in the forearm and back muscles during laparoscopic surgery. Surg Laparosc Endosc Percutan Tech 2013; 23: 203–7.

[30] Szeto GPY, Ho P, Ting CW, Poon JTC, Tsang RCC, Cheng SWK. A study of surgeons' postural muscle activity during open, laparoscopic, and endovascular surgery. Surg Endosc 2010; 24: 1712–21.

[31] Büchel D, Mårvik R, Hallabrin B, Matern U. Ergonomics of disposable handles for minimally invasive surgery. Surg Endosc 2010; 24: 992–1004.

[32] Fan Y, Kong G, Meng Y, Tan S, Wei K, Zhang Q, et al. Comparative assessment of surgeons' task performance and surgical ergonomics associated with conventional and modified flank positions: a simulation study. Surg Endosc 2014; 28: 3249–56.

[33] Wilson MR, Poolton JM, Malhotra N, Ngo K, Bright E, Masters RSW. Development and validation of a surgical workload measure: the surgery task load index (SURG-TLX). World J Surg 2011; 35: 1961–9.

[34] Abdelrahman AM, Bingener J, Yu D, Lowndes BR, Mohamed A, McConico AL, et al. Impact of single-incision laparoscopic cholecystectomy (SILC) versus conventional laparoscopic cholecystectomy (CLC) procedures on surgeon stress and workload: a randomized controlled trial. Surg Endosc 2016; 30: 1205–11.

[35] Hu JSL, Lu J, Tan WB, Lomanto D. Training improves laparoscopic tasks performance and decreases operator workload. Surg Endosc 2016; 30: 1742–6.

[36] Liang B, Qi L, Yang J, Cao Z, Zu X, Liu L, Wang L. Ergonomic status of laparoscopic urologic surgery: survey results from 241 urologic surgeons in china. PLoS One 2013; 8(7): e70423.

[37] Cass GK, Vyas S, Akande V. Prolonged laparoscopic surgery is associated with an increased risk of vertebral disc prolapse. J Obstet Gynaecol 2014; 34(1): 74–8.

[38] Franasiak J, Ko EM, Kidd J, Secord AA, Bell M, Boggess JF, Gehrig PA. Physical strain and urgent need for ergonomic training among gynecologic oncologists who perform minimally invasive surgery. Gynecol Oncol 2012; 126(3): 437–42.

[39] Sutton E, Irvin M, Zeigler C, Lee G, Park A. The ergonomics of women in surgery. Surg Endosc 2014; 28(4): 1051–5.

[40] Lucas-Hernández M, Pagador JB, Pérez-Duarte FJ, Castelló P, Sánchez-Margallo FM. Ergonomics problems due to the use and design of dissector and needle holder. Surg Laparosc Endosc Percutan Tech 2014; 24: e170–7.

[41] Filisetti C, Cho A, Riccipetitoni G, Saxena AK. Analysis of hand size and ergonomics of instruments in pediatric minimally invasive surgery. Surg Laparosc Endosc Percutan Tech 2015; 25(5): e159–62.

[42] Nieboer TE, Massa M, Weinans MJN, Vierhout ME, Kluivers KB, Stegeman DF. Does training of the nondominant upper extremity reduce the surgeon's muscular strain during laparoscopy?: Results from a randomized controlled trial. Surg Innov 2013; 20: 292–8.

[43] Haramis G, Rosales JC, Palacios JM, Okhunov Z, Mues AC, Lee D, et al. Prospective randomized evaluation of FOOT gel pads for operating room staff COMFORT during laparoscopic renal surgery. Urology 2010; 76: 1405–8.

[44] Yurko YY, Scerbo MW, Prabhu AS, Acker CE, Stefanidis D. Higher mental workload is associated with poorer laparoscopic performance as measured by the NASA-TLX tool. Simul Healthc 2010; 5(5): 267–71.

[45] Riggle JD, Miller EE, McCrory B, Meitl A, Lim E, Hallbeck MS, et al. Ergonomic comparison of laparoscopic hand instruments in a single site surgery simulator with novices. Minim Invasive Ther Allied Technol 2015; 24: 68–76.

[46] Bertolaccini L, Viti A, Terzi A. Ergon-trial: ergonomic evaluation of single-port access versus three-port access video-assisted thoracic surgery. Surg Endosc 2015; 29: 2934–40.

[47] Aubdoollah TH. Clinical outcomes and ergonomics analysis of three laparoscopic techniques for Hirschsprung's disease. World J Gastroenterol 2015; 21: 8903.

[48] Tsai Y-C, Lin VC-H, Chung S-D, Ho C-H, Jaw F-S, Tai H-C. Ergonomic and geometric tricks of laparoendoscopic single-site surgery (LESS) by using conventional laparoscopic instruments. Surg Endosc 2012; 26: 2671–7.

[49] Lee GI, Lee MR, Clanton T, Clanton T, Sutton E, Park AE, et al. Comparative assessment of physical and cognitive ergonomics associated with robotic and traditional laparoscopic surgeries. Surg Endosc 2014; 28: 456–65.

[50] Stefanidis D, Wang F, Korndorffer JR, Dunne JB, Scott DJ. Robotic assistance improves intracorporeal suturing performance and safety in the operating room while decreasing operator workload. Surg Endosc 2010; 24: 377–82.

[51] Moore LJ, Wilson MR, McGrath JS, Waine E, Masters RSW, Vine SJ. Surgeons' display reduced mental effort and workload while performing robotically assisted surgical tasks, when compared to conventional laparoscopy. Surg Endosc 2015; 29: 2553–60.

[52] Passerotti CC, Franco F, Bissoli JCC, Tiseo B, Oliveira CM, Buchalla CAO, et al. Comparison of the learning curves and frustration level in performing laparoscopic and robotic training skills by experts and novices. Int Urol Nephrol 2015; 47: 1075–84.

[53] Rousek JB, Brown-Clerk B, Lowndes BR, Balogh BJ, Hallbeck MS. Optimizing integration of electrosurgical hand controls within a laparoscopic surgical tool. Minim Invasive Ther Allied Technol 2012; 21: 222–33.

[54] Steinhilber B, Seibt R, Reiff F, Rieger MA, Kraemer B, Rothmund R. Effect of a laparoscopic instrument with rotatable handle piece on biomechanical stress during laparoscopic procedures. Surg Endosc 2016; 30: 78–88.

[55] Yu D, Lowndes B, Morrow M, Kaufman K, Bingener J, Hallbeck S. Impact of novel shift handle laparoscopic tool on wrist ergonomics and task performance. Surg Endosc 2015. [Epub ahead of print].

[56] Di Lorenzo N, Camperchioli I, Gaspari AL. Radius surgical system and conventional laparoscopic instruments in abdominal surgery: application, learning curve and ergonomy. Surg Oncol 2007;16(Suppl 1): S69–72.

[57] Hirano Y, Inaki N, Ishikawa N, Watanabe G. Laparoscopic treatment for esophageal achalasia and gastro-esophago-reflex disease using radius surgical system. Indian J Surg 2013; 75: 160–2.

[58] Gözen AS, Tokas T, Tschada A, Jalal A, Klein J, Rassweiler J. Direct comparison of the different conventional laparoscopic positions with the ethos surgical platform in a laparoscopic pelvic surgery simulation setting. J Endourol 2015; 29: 95–9.

[59] Steinhilber B, Hoffmann S, Karlovic K, Pfeffer S, Maier T, Hallasheh O, et al. Development of an arm support system to improve ergonomics in laparoscopic surgery: study design and provisional results. Surg Endosc 2015; 29: 2851–8.

[60] Xiao D, Jakimowicz JJ, Albayrak A, Buzink SN, Botden SMBI, Goossens RHM. Face, content, and construct validity of a novel portable ergonomic simulator for basic laparoscopic skills. J Surg Educ 2014; 71: 65–72.

2

Laparoscopic Surgery for Gastric Cancer

Talha Sarigoz, Inanc Samil Sarici, Ozgul Duzgun and
Mustafa Uygar Kalayci

Abstract

In patients with gastric cancer, surgical resection is the only treatment that can offer cure
or increase long-term survival. With the accumulation of experience in laparoscopic radical gastrectomy and the progress in surgical instruments, laparoscopic surgery for gastric
cancer has gained popularity despite initial concerns regarding safety and oncological
adequacy. As a result, laparoscopic technique has been widely applied in gastric cancer.
Different meta-analyses showed that laparoscopic procedures are associated with less
blood loss but longer operation time. Many studies have reported outcomes of laparoscopic surgery for early gastric cancer, but several authors also have shown that a laparoscopic approach can also be used in cases of advanced gastric cancer. We therefore
conducted this study to expand our experience and to evaluate laparoscopic gastrectomy
step by step in the light of recent reports while defining key points and surgical technique.

Keywords: laparoscopic surgery, gastric cancer, gastrectomy, lymphadenectomy,
advanced, early gastric cancer, laparoscopic gastrectomy

1. Introduction

Gastric cancer (GC) is the fifth most common malignancy and the third most common cause
of cancer-related deaths worldwide in both sexes combined [1]. Surgery with either total or
subtotal gastrectomy and lymphadenectomy is the initial treatment [2]. The first example of
gastrectomy for cancer was described by Theodor Billroth and the first laparoscopy-assisted
gastrectomy was performed by Kitano et al. in 1991 for a patient with early GC [3, 4]. In the
last two decades, in parallel to advances in surgical devices and technical expertise, minimally
invasive surgery has become the new trend and the laparoscopy has increasingly started
being applied for GC as an alternative to open surgery. However, due to complexity of the
lymph node structure and contiguity of stomach to gross vascular structures, it is technically

demanding. During the procedure, it is equally important to ensure adequate resection and pay attention to some precautions [5]. In this chapter, we will clarify pre-operative approach, technical considerations as well as clinical outcomes of laparoscopic surgery (LS) for GC based on the recent reports in the literature.

2. Preoperative approach

2.1. Indications for laparoscopic surgery

Most of the reports evaluated early GC population and common consensus is that laparoscopic gastrectomy is appropriate for early-stage GC with benefits of reduced need for painkillers, early discharge, rapid recovery of bowel movement, less pulmonary function disorders, and better cosmetic results [5, 6]. There is agreement about performing laparoscopic total gastrectomy for proximal GC with T1 N0 disease and laparoscopic distal gastrectomy for distal GC with T1–2 N0 disease [5]. Regarding advanced stage cancers, there is still debate over appropriateness of laparoscopy concerning oncologic adequacy of lymphadenectomy with tumor-free margins. Recent meta-analysis and cohorts demonstrated favorable short- and long-term outcomes of laparoscopic gastrectomy for advanced stage GC; but in order to recommend it as an alternative to open surgery, there is still room for prospective clinical trials and longer-follow-up studies [7–9].

2.2. Determination of resection margin

Lack of tactile feedback limits assessment of the tumor during laparoscopic surgery. Since laparoscopic gastrectomy has been performed mostly for early GC and achieving tumor-free margins is important in terms of oncological principles, different methods have been proposed for safe determination of resection line in tumors without serosal surface invasion. Reported various procedures include preoperative or intraoperative endoscopic dye injection, preoperative endoscopic clipping along with intraoperative endoscopy, intraoperative radiography or ultrasonography [10–14]. None of these methods has wide acceptance and choice of technique vary with institution.

2.3. Nutritional status of patients

As gastric cancer is a serious malignancy of the upper intestinal tract, patients are at risk for malnutrition due to maldigestion and malabsorption. On the other hand, surgery itself imposes protein and energy requirements and it can aggravate pre-existing nutritional disorders [15]. There is a lack of clinical evidence about role of laparoscopic gastrectomy in malnourished patients with GC. A recent retrospective study reported significantly less postoperative complications and faster recovery for laparoscopic gastrectomy compared to open surgery [16]. But, prospective clinical trials to analyze short- and long-term effects of preoperative nutritional support, chemotherapy and dissection type are required to recommend laparoscopic gastrectomy for malnourished patients.

2.4. Presence of enlarged lymph nodes in preoperative imaging

There are controversies on the extent of lymphadenectomy for GC. Nevertheless, lymph node dissection is recommended for staging and prevention of local recurrence. Most of the patients with GC are diagnosed at a later stage of the disease, often with enlarged lymph nodes. Since lymphadenectomy is a challenging procedure, especially in laparoscopic setting, enlarged nodes interfere with anatomical structures and disrupt the course of the dissection. In a late retrospective study, performing laparoscopic gastrectomy for GC with pre-operative enlarged lymph nodes was found to be safe and effective [17]. Yet, these results should be supported with prospective research to make recommendation.

2.5. Obese patients

Obese patients carry high risk for comorbid diseases and they are directly associated with intra- and post-operative complications [18]. Obesity was considered as a relative contraindication for laparoscopy, but with the advances in laparoscopic equipment and growing experience, initial studies with laparoscopic surgery in obese patients have shown promise [19]. According to the reports in the literature, due to abundant visceral fat content and difficult manipulation of tissue, operation times in laparoscopic gastrectomy were longer compared to open surgery [20, 21]. Not only obesity, but also high body mass index (BMI ≥ 25 kg/m^2) was shown to affect operation time and retrieved lymph node number negatively [22]. On the other hand, the 5-year survival rates of patients who underwent laparoscopic gastrectomy and open gastrectomy were similar [23]. But regarding early post-operative outcomes, we cannot mention that there is an agreement [20, 21, 23]. Despite negative findings, laparoscopic gastrectomy is likely to be the choice of surgery in obese patients with growing experience.

2.6. Elderly patients

In parallel to increasing age, functional capacity decreases at some point and this situation creates risk for surgery. Considering advantages, elderly may benefit from laparoscopic surgery. In an updated pooled meta-analysis, laparoscopic gastrectomy was found to reduce surgery-related cardiopulmonary disease and also better cognitive outcomes were observed compared to open surgery [24]. But, lack of randomized controlled studies in the literature prevent from making precise conclusions.

3. Technical considerations

3.1. The importance of lymphadenectomy in gastric cancer

Lymph node metastasis (LNM) is the most common pattern of metastatic spread in gastric cancer [25]. The reported frequency of LNM in gastric cancer can be seen up to 80%. Lymphatic networks are plenty in the layer of the gastric wall, particularly in the submucosa and serosa, which simplify metastasis. Oncological outcomes will not be reached if gastrectomy alone is performed for gastric cancer. Therefore, lymphatic flow of the stomach and characteristics of metastasis have been continuously examined by researchers. In the Japanese gastric cancer treatment guidelines based on the third English edition of the Japanese Classification of Gastric Carcinoma and the Japanese Gastric Cancer Association defined the extent of systematic lymphadenectomy according to the type of gastrectomy indicated [26]. Lymph node metastasis in gastric cancer is usually associated with the location of the tumor, and metastasis follows the lymphatic drainage routes from the superficial to the profoundus. For this reason, lymph nodes are numbered and dissection for functional lymph node resection was defined. Laparoscopic gastrectomy, which begins with D1 dissection in early gastric cancer treatment, can now be done easily with the aid of technology (laparoscopy, robotic surgery) and D2 dissection technique is routinely performed in the treatment of advanced GC [27] (**Tables 1** and **2**).

3.2. Surgical technique of laparoscopic gastrectomy with D2 lymphadenectomy

3.2.1. Patient's position and location of trocars

The patient is placed in the modified lithotomy position. The surgical table is adjusted 20–30° into the reverse Trendelenburg position. The surgeon stands on the patient's leg, the assistant is on the right side, and the camera operator is between the patient's left side. Besides routine laparoscopic devices, advance vessel sealing systems, all types of intestinal Endo-GIA and circular staplers must be available on the operating table. The intervention generally performed by using five ports. Additionally, subxiphoid sixth port can be required during the splenic hilar lymph node dissection. 10-mm optic port is placed 1 cm above the umbilicus. 15-mm trocar left preaxillary and 5 mm trocar right preaxillary is inserted in the line 2 cm below the costal margin. Two 5-mm ports are placed bilaterally in each hypochondrium for assisting and dissection purposes (**Figure 1**).

3.2.2. Surgical procedure

Laparoscopic exploration is used for preoperative staging, liver and peritoneal metastasis which can reduce unnecessary laparotomies. Once it is determined that it is suitable for surgery, the procedure continues in four steps as left part region, right part region, cardiac region, and reconstruction (**Table 3**).

3.2.2.1. Left part region (4sa, 4sv, 10, 11d)

The approach for removing the greater omentum begins from the superior border of the transverse colon. After that, the division is extended toward the flexura of left and the right colon. In the continuation of the dissection, splenic ligaments must be separated due to prevent of iatrogenic splenic injury which may be caused by traction. Gastrosplenic, splenocolic, splenorenal, and splenophrenic ligaments need to be separated in this stage. The omentectomy helps to achieve a lymphadenectomy corresponding to lymph node stations 4sa and 4sv according to the Japanese classification. The left gastro-omental vessels are perfectly identified clipped and divided. After this dissection, the short gastric vessels will be divided using the sealing

Regional lymph nodes of stomach

1. Right cardia lymph nodes

2. Left cardia lymph nodes

3. Lymph nodes along the lesser curvature

4. Lymph nodes along the greater curvature

    •   Station **4sa:** lymph nodes along the short gastric vessels

    •   Station **4sb:** lymph nodes along the left gastroepiploic vessels

    •   Station **4d:** lymph nodes along the right gastroepiploic vessel

5. Suprapyloric group of lymph nodes or nodes along the right gastric artery

6. Infrapyloric groups of lymph nodes

7. Lymph nodes along the left gastric artery

8. Lymph nodes along the common hepatic artery

    •   Station **8a:** anterosuperior group

    •   Station **8b:** posterior group

9. Lymph nodes around the celiac artery

10. Lymph nodes at the splenic hilum

11. Lymph nodes along the splenic artery

    •   Station **11p:** along the proximal splenic artery

    •   Station **11d:** along the distal splenic artery

12. Lymph nodes in the hepatoduodenal ligament

    •   Station **12a:** along the hepatic artery

    •   Station **12b:** along the bile duct

    •   Station **12p:** behind the portal vein

13. Lymph nodes behind the pancreatic head

14. Lymph nodes at the root of the mesentery or the SMA

15. Lymph nodes along the middle colic artery

16. Para-aortic group of lymph nodes

    •   Station **16a1:** lymph node in the aortic hiatus

    •   Station **16a2:** lymph node around the abdominal aorta (from the upper margin of the celiac trunk to the lower margin of the left renal vein)

    •   Station **16b1:** lymph node around the abdominal aorta (from the lower margin of the left renal vein to the upper margin of the inferior mesenteric artery)

    •   Station **16b2:** lymph node around the abdominal aorta (from the upper margin of the inferior mesenteric artery to the aortic bifurcation)

Table 1. Numbering lymph nodes according to the Japanese Research Society for Gastric Cancer.

D0	No dissection or incomplete dissection of the Group 1 nodes
D1	Dissection of all the Group 1 nodes (No.1–6 lymph nodes)
D2	Dissection of all the Group 1 and Group 2 nodes (D1 station + No.7–11 lymph nodes)
D3	Dissection of all the Group 1, Group 2 and Group 3 nodes (D2+ No. 12–16 lymph nodes)

Table 2. Definitions of lymphadenectomy in gastric cancer.

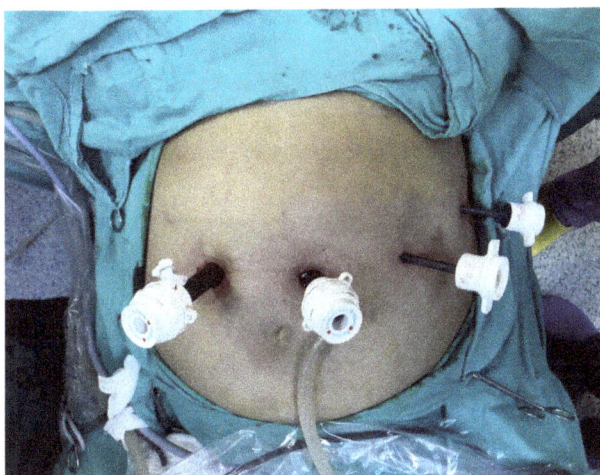

Figure 1. Patient's position and location of trocars.

1	Left part region (4sa, 4sv, 10, 11d)
2	Right part region (4d, 5, 6, 7, 8a, 8p, 9, 11p, 12a, 12b, 12p)
3	Cardiac region [1–3]
4	Gastric resection and reconstruction

Table 3. Steps of laparoscopic gastrectomy for gastric cancer.

systems. This dissection should be continued until the left crus of the diaphragm clearly seen. At this time, the lymph node 10 and 11d in the splenic hilus is gently excised (**Figures 2** and **3**).

3.2.2.2. Right part region (4d, 5, 6, 7, 8a, 8p, 9, 11p, 12a, 12b, 12p)

The dissection is then continued toward the right part of the abdomen. Dissection of the gastro-omental ligament is pursued in this area. This dissection allows to drop the right colon and to access the duodenum. This maneuver also allows to expose the anterior aspect of the pancreatic head and to access the right gastro-omental pedicle, where a lymphadenectomy should be performed in order to control lymph node station 6 (**Figure 4**).

Right gastro-omental vessels are dissected, isolated, and divided. Once this first mobilization and 6-station of lymphadenectomy step has been performed, the first portion of the duodenum will be dissected and isolated, prior to moving on to the supragastric compartment. The common bile duct, hepatic artery, and portal vein, which form the hepatoduodenal ligament,

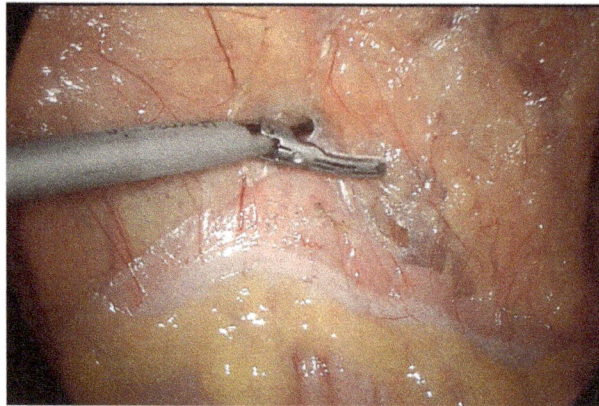

Figure 2. Lift of transvers colon and dissection of anterior transvers mesocolon fascia.

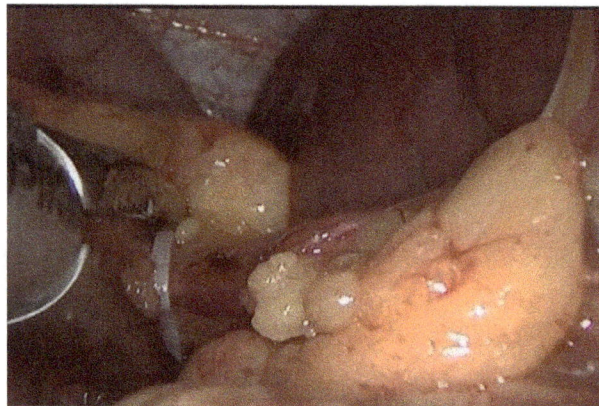

Figure 3. The left gastro-omental vessel is clipped and divided.

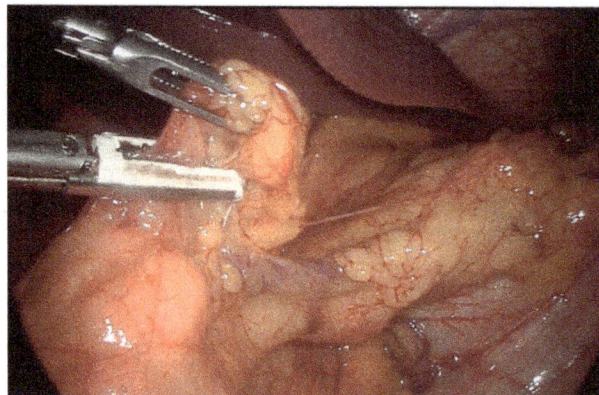

Figure 4. Dissection of number 6 lymphatic area.

are identified. The right gastric artery will also be identified and divided along with lymph node dissection at the level of lymph node station 5. The 12a, 12b, and 12p lymph node stations in the hepatoduodenal ligament are excised with vessel sealing devices (**Figure 5**).

Duodenal division is then performed approximately 2 cm distally from the pylorus by Endo-GIA blue cartridge. After dissection of the hepatic proper artery, resection will be carried on at the superior border of the pancreas at the level of the common hepatic artery, namely lymph node

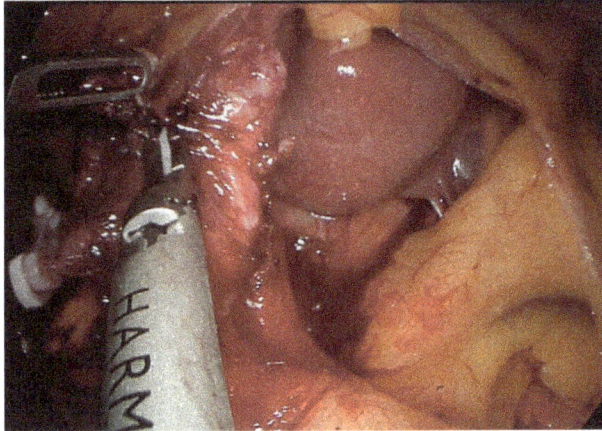

Figure 5. Dissection of hepatoduodenal lymphatic area.

stations 8 and 9. The left coronary vein is also identified, clipped, and divided. Dissection is pursued toward the coeliac trunk with lymph node dissection of stations 9. Dissection of the left gastric artery is begun along with lymph node dissection of station 7. The left gastric artery is clipped and divided. After that 11p lymph node stations along the splenic artery are excised. Care should be taken during dissection due to the tortuous structure of splenic artery (**Figures 6** and **7**).

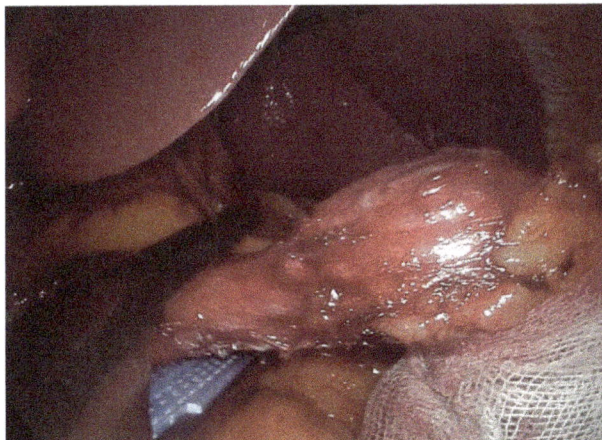

Figure 6. Transection of duodenum.

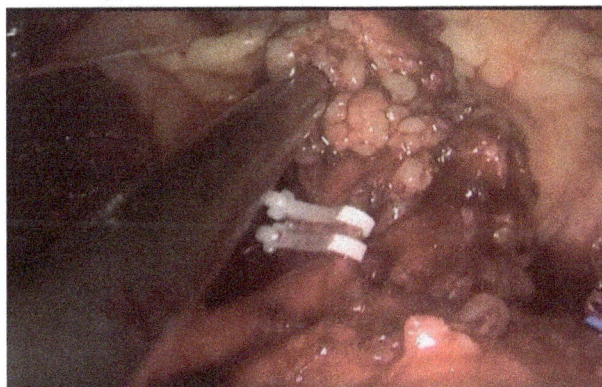

Figure 7. Dissection of number 7, 8, and 9 lymphatic area.

3.2.2.3. Cardiac region

The lymph nodes in the cardiac region are located on both sides of the cardia and along the lesser curvature [1–3]. Hepatogastric ligament is opened by vessel sealing devices in the avascular area at the posterior wall of the gastric lesser curvature. Thus, the gastric lesser curvature is fully bared and dissection of the No. 3 lymph nodes is done. The left and right diaphragm crus are identified and the phrenoesophageal membrane is dissected. Lymph nodes No:1 and No:2 are excised. The abdominal part of the esophagus is bared 5 cm in the abdomen. Left and right vagal nerves divided (**Figure 8**).

3.2.2.4. Gastric resection and reconstruction

The reconstruction should be in different forms according to the extent of the resection. Proximal resection was performed with Endo GIA blue cartridge which is placed from 15 mm trocar. Trans oral OrVil™ (Covidien Mansfield, USA) is propagated from the esophagus and anvil is placed in the esophageal stump. Transvers mesocolon lifted and the small window open from the avascular area. Jejunal ans is divided at 20 cm from the Treitz ligament by Endo GIA blue cartridge. Esophagojejunostomy is done with 25 mm circular stapler if totally gastrectomy planned or gastrojejunostomy is performed with EndoGIA if subtotal gastrectomy intended. Jejunal stump is closed with Endo GIA blue cartridge. Laparoscopic reinforcement

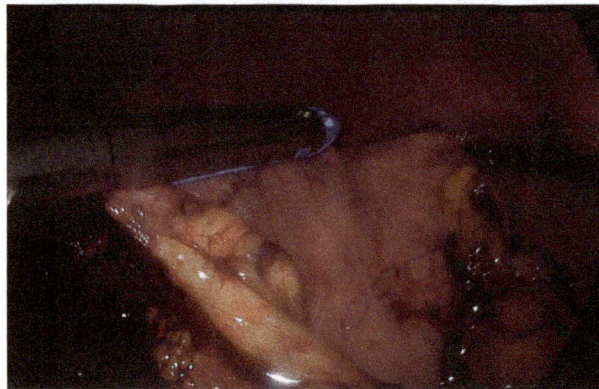

Figure 8. Dissection of cardiac lymphatic area.

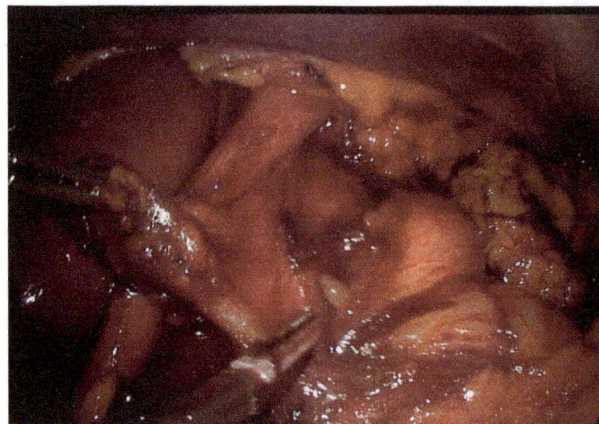

Figure 9. Proximal resection of stomach with EndoGIA.

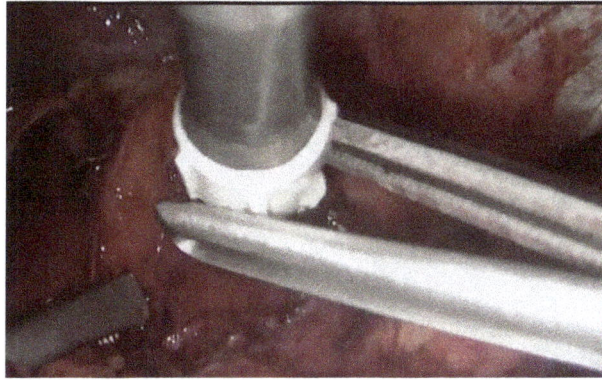

Figure 10. OrVil™ placement in the esophageal stump.

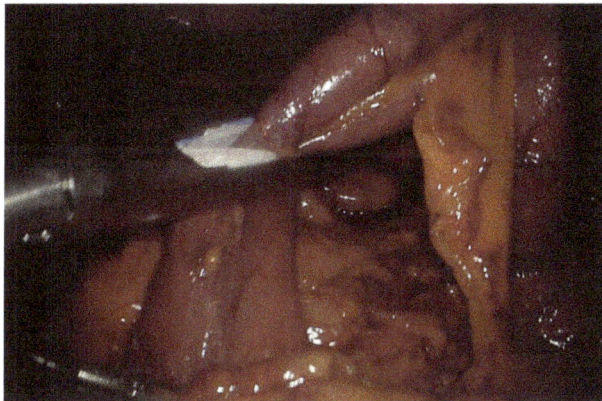

Figure 11. Division of jejunal ans 20 cm distal to the Treitz ligament.

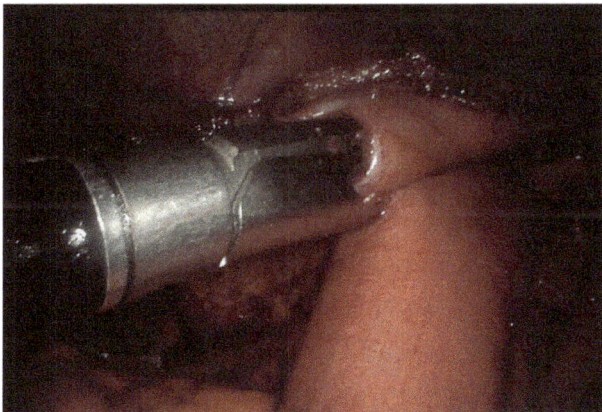

Figure 12. Gastrojejunostomy with EndoGIA.

sutures can be added if needed. Jejunum is fixed to the diaphragm crus. The jejunojejunostomy is also performed by means of a side to side Endo GIA blue cartridge stapler. Placement of the gastric tube is controlled laparoscopically. This tube is lowered until the distal part of the alimentary limb. A wound protector is placed into the defect, hence allowing for the extraction of the entire specimen, including the whole stomach and the omentum (**Figures 9–13, Table 4**).

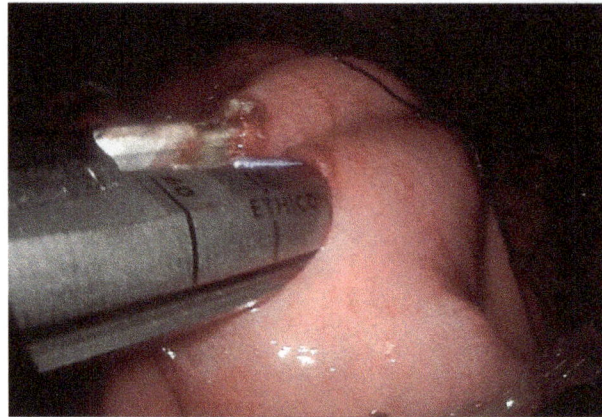

Figure 13. Jejunojejunostomy with EndoGIA.

Subtotal gastrectomy	Total gastrectomy
• Totally laparoscopic gastroduodenostomy (Billroth 1)	• Roux-en-Y esophagojejunostomy
• Billroth 1 through mini laparotomy	• Hand-sewn anastomosis
• Billroth 1 with hand port	• Laparoscopic
• Roux-en-Y Gastrojejunostomy	• Mini-laparotomy
	• Mechanical anastomosis
	• Circular stapler
	• Manually loaded anvil
	• Transoral (OrVil™)

Table 4. Different reconstruction forms according to the resection types.

4. Post-operative outcomes

4.1. Early post-operative outcomes

Initial studies with laparoscopic gastrectomy consisted of mostly early GC and with growing experience it has been started to apply to later stages of the disease. Laparoscopic gastrectomy whether performed for early or advanced GC has advantages such as less blood loss, early ambulation, rapid recovery of bowel movement, and shorter hospitalization compared to open surgery [28–31]. Complication rates of laparoscopic gastrectomy for early GC ranged from 4.2 to 23.3% and these results did not differ from open surgery [29, 32–34]. In the latest ongoing clinical trials, short-term results have been shared. While, laparoscopic surgery for advanced GC has a complication rate of 16.4%, it is 24.3% for open surgery [35–37]. These studies will be finalized in 2018. In an ongoing study in Japan, short-term results have revealed incidence of anastomotic leakage rate as 4.7% for laparoscopic surgery in advanced stage [37]. In the retrospective studies, anastomotic leakage rate during LS for advanced GC was reported to range from 1.1 to 2.7% [30, 38–40]. But this risk should be evaluated appropriately.

4.2. Late post-operative outcomes

According to single-center studies, after laparoscopic gastrectomy for early GC, the morbidity rates ranged from 10 to 14.8% and mortality rates from 0 to 1.1% [6, 41, 42]. Regarding laparoscopic gastrectomy for AGC, the morbidity rates ranged from 8.0 to 24.2% but there was no significant difference compared to open surgery [30, 39, 40]. There are ongoing randomized phase-II and III studies in Asian Countries. They are expected to give scientifically more reliable results [30, 35]. Initial results indicate that LS for advanced GC is feasible and safe but surgeon experience and institution volume play important role on patient outcome. Long-term outcomes should be clarified with well-established studies.

Author details

Talha Sarigoz[1]*, Inanc Samil Sarici[2], Ozgul Duzgun[3] and Mustafa Uygar Kalayci[4]

*Address all correspondence to: sarigozt.md@gmail.com

1 Department of General Surgery, Sason State Hospital, Batman, Turkey

2 Department of General Surgery, Kanuni Sultan Suleyman Training and Research Hospital, Istanbul, Turkey

3 Division of Surgical Oncology, Department of General Surgery, Umraniye Training and Research Hospital, Istanbul, Turkey

4 Department of General Surgery, Kanuni Sultan Suleyman Training and Research Hospital, Istanbul, Turkey

References

[1] Global Burden of Disease Cancer C, Fitzmaurice C, Allen C, Barber RM, Barregard L, Bhutta ZA, et al. Global, regional, and national cancer incidence, mortality, years of life lost, years lived with disability, and disability-adjusted life-years for 32 cancer groups, 1990 to 2015: A systematic analysis for the global burden of disease study. JAMA Oncology. 2017;**3**(4):524-548

[2] Lutz MP, Zalcberg JR, Ducreux M, Ajani JA, Allum W, Aust D, et al. Highlights of the EORTC St. Gallen International Expert Consensus on the primary therapy of gastric, gastroesophageal and oesophageal cancer—Differential treatment strategies for subtypes of early gastroesophageal cancer. European Journal of Cancer. 2012;**48**(16):2941-2953

[3] Kitano S, Iso Y, Moriyama M, Sugimachi K. Laparoscopy-assisted Billroth I Gastrectomy. Surgical Laparoscopy & Endoscopy. 1994;**4**(2):146-148

[4] Billroth T. Offenes schreiben an Herr, Dr. L. Wittelshofer. Wiener Medizinische Wochenschrift. 1881;**26**:731

[5] Brar S, Law C, McLeod R, Helyer L, Swallow C, Paszat L, et al. Defining surgical quality in gastric cancer: A RAND/UCLA appropriateness study. Journal of the American College of Surgeons. 2013;**217**(2):347-357. e1

[6] Kitano S, Shiraishi N, Fujii K, Yasuda K, Inomata M, Adachi YA. Randomized controlled trial comparing open vs laparoscopy-assisted distal gastrectomy for the treatment of early gastric cancer: An interim report. Surgery. 2002;**131**(1 Suppl):S306-S311

[7] Son T, Hyung WJ, Lee JH, Kim YM, Noh SH. Minimally invasive surgery for serosa-positive gastric cancer (pT4a) in patients with preoperative diagnosis of cancer without serosal invasion. Surgical Endoscopy. 2014;**28**(3):866-874

[8] Lee J, Kim W. Long-term outcomes after laparoscopy-assisted gastrectomy for advanced gastric cancer: Analysis of consecutive 106 experiences. Journal of Surgical Oncology. 2009;**100**(8):693-698

[9] Huscher CG, Mingoli A, Sgarzini G, Brachini G, Binda B, Di Paola M, et al. Totally laparoscopic total and subtotal gastrectomy with extended lymph node dissection for early and advanced gastric cancer: Early and long-term results of a 100-patient series. American Journal of Surgery. 2007;**194**(6):839-844. discussion 44

[10] Xuan Y, Hur H, Byun CS, Han SU, Cho YK. Efficacy of intraoperative gastroscopy for tumor localization in totally laparoscopic distal gastrectomy for cancer in the middle third of the stomach. Surgical Endoscopy. 2013;**27**(11):4364-4370

[11] Park DJ, Lee HJ, Kim SG, Jung HC, Song IS, Lee KU, et al. Intraoperative gastroscopy for gastric surgery. Surgical Endoscopy. 2005;**19**(10):1358-1361

[12] Nakagawa M, Ehara K, Ueno M, Tanaka T, Kaida S, Udagawa H. Accurate, safe, and rapid method of intraoperative tumor identification for totally laparoscopic distal gastrectomy: Injection of mixed fluid of sodium hyaluronate and patent blue. Surgical Endoscopy. 2014;**28**(4):1371-1375

[13] Kim HI, Hyung WJ, Lee CR, Lim JS, An JY, Cheong JH, et al. Intraoperative portable abdominal radiograph for tumor localization: A simple and accurate method for laparoscopic gastrectomy. Surgical Endoscopy. 2011;**25**(3):958-963

[14] Kawakatsu S, Ohashi M, Hiki N, Nunobe S, Nagino M, Sano T. Use of endoscopy to determine the resection margin during laparoscopic gastrectomy for cancer. The British Journal of Surgery. 2017

[15] Mariette C, De Botton ML, Piessen G. Surgery in esophageal and gastric cancer patients: What is the role for nutrition support in your daily practice? Annals of Surgical Oncology. 2012;**19**(7):2128-2134

[16] Zheng HL, Lu J, Zheng CH, Li P, Xie JW, Wang JB, et al. Short- and long-term outcomes in malnourished patients after laparoscopic or open radical gastrectomy. World Journal of Surgery. 2017

[17] Chen QY, Huang CM, Zheng CH, Li P, Xie JW, Wang JB, et al. Do preoperative enlarged lymph nodes affect the oncologic outcome of laparoscopic radical gastrectomy for gastric cancer? Oncotarget. 2017;8(5):8825-8834

[18] Tjeertes EK, Hoeks SE, Beks SB, Valentijn TM, Hoofwijk AG, Stolker RJ. Obesity—A risk factor for postoperative complications in general surgery? BMC Anesthesiology. 2015;15:112

[19] Loffer FD, Pent D. Laparoscopy in the obese patient. American Journal of Obstetrics and Gynecology. 1976;125(1):104-107

[20] Yasuda K, Inomata M, Shiraishi N, Izumi K, Ishikawa K, Kitano S. Laparoscopy-assisted distal gastrectomy for early gastric cancer in obese and nonobese patients. Surgical Endoscopy. 2004;18(8):1253-1256

[21] Kim MG, Yook JH, Kim KC, Kim TH, Kim HS, Kim BS, et al. Influence of obesity on early surgical outcomes of laparoscopic-assisted gastrectomy in gastric cancer. Surgical Laparoscopy, Endoscopy & Percutaneous Techniques. 2011;21(3):151-154

[22] Lee HJ, Kim HH, Kim MC, Ryu SY, Kim W, Song KY, et al. The impact of a high body mass index on laparoscopy assisted gastrectomy for gastric cancer. Surgical Endoscopy. 2009;23(11):2473-2479

[23] Son SY, Jung DH, Lee CM, Ahn SH, Ahn HS, Park DJ, et al. Laparoscopic gastrectomy versus open gastrectomy for gastric cancer in patients with body mass index of 30 kg/m^2 or more. Surgical Endoscopy. 2015;29(8):2126-2132

[24] Zong L, Wu A, Wang W, Deng J, Aikou S, Yamashita H, et al. Feasibility of laparoscopic gastrectomy for elderly gastric cancer patients: Meta-analysis of non-randomized controlled studies. Oncotarget. 2017;8(31):51878-51887

[25] Huang C-M, Zheng C-H. Summary of anatomy and physiology of perigastric lymphatic system. In: Huang C-M, Zheng C-H, editors. Laparoscopic Gastrectomy for Gastric Cancer: Surgical Technique and Lymphadenectomy. Dordrecht: Springer Netherlands; 2015. pp. 1-6

[26] Japanese Gastric Cancer A. Japanese gastric cancer treatment guidelines 2010 (ver. 3). Gastric Cancer. 2011;14(2):113-123

[27] RH T, Li P, Xie JW, Wang JB, Lin JX, Lu J, et al. Development of lymph node dissection in laparoscopic gastrectomy: Safety and technical tips. Transl. Gastroenterología y Hepatología. 2017;2:23

[28] Kim YW, Baik YH, Yun YH, Nam BH, Kim DH, Choi IJ, et al. Improved quality of life outcomes after laparoscopy-assisted distal gastrectomy for early gastric cancer: Results of a prospective randomized clinical trial. Annals of Surgery. 2008;248(5):721-727

[29] Kim HH, Hyung WJ, Cho GS, Kim MC, Han SU, Kim W, et al. Morbidity and mortality of laparoscopic gastrectomy versus open gastrectomy for gastric cancer: An interim report—A phase III multicenter, prospective, randomized trial (KLASS trial). Annals of Surgery. 2010;251(3):417-420

[30] Hu Y, Huang C, Sun Y, Su X, Cao H, Hu J, et al. Morbidity and mortality of laparo-scopic versus open D2 distal Gastrectomy for advanced gastric cancer: A randomized controlled trial. Journal of Clinical Oncology. 2016;**34**(12):1350-1357

[31] Hayashi H, Ochiai T, Shimada H, Gunji Y. Prospective randomized study of open versus laparoscopy-assisted distal gastrectomy with extraperigastric lymph node dissection for early gastric cancer. Surgical Endoscopy. 2005;**19**(9):1172-1176

[32] Lee JH, Han HS, Lee JHA. Prospective randomized study comparing open vs laparos-copy-assisted distal gastrectomy in early gastric cancer: Early results. Surgical Endos-copy. 2005;**19**(2):168-173

[33] Hosono S, Arimoto Y, Ohtani H, Kanamiya Y. Meta-analysis of short-term outcomes after laparoscopy-assisted distal gastrectomy. World Journal of Gastroenterology. 2006; **12**(47):7676-7683

[34] Adachi Y, Shiraishi N, Shiromizu A, Bandoh T, Aramaki M, Kitano S. Laparoscopy-assisted Billroth I gastrectomy compared with conventional open gastrectomy. Archives of Surgery. 2000;**135**(7):806-810

[35] Lee H-J, Hyung WJ, Yang H-K, Han SU, Park Y-K, An JY, et al. Morbidity of laparoscopic distal gastrectomy with D2 lymphadenectomy compared with open distal gastrectomy for locally advanced gastric cancer: Short term outcomes from multicenter randomized controlled trial (KLASS-02). Journal of Clinical Oncology. 2016;**34**(15_suppl):4062

[36] Kinoshita T, Kaito A. Current status and future perspectives of laparoscopic radical sur-gery for advanced gastric cancer. Transl. Gastroenterología y Hepatología. 2017;**2**:43

[37] Inaki N, Etoh T, Ohyama T, Uchiyama K, Katada N, Koeda K, et al. A multi-institu-tional, prospective, phase II feasibility study of laparoscopy-assisted distal gastrectomy with D2 lymph node dissection for locally advanced gastric cancer (JLSSG0901). World Journal of Surgery. 2015;**39**(11):2734-2741

[38] Kim W, Song KY, Lee HJ, Han SU, Hyung WJ, Cho GS. The impact of comorbidity on surgical outcomes in laparoscopy-assisted distal gastrectomy: A retrospective analysis of multicenter results. Annals of Surgery. 2008;**248**(5):793-799

[39] Shinohara T, Satoh S, Kanaya S, Ishida Y, Taniguchi K, Isogaki J, et al. Laparoscopic versus open D2 gastrectomy for advanced gastric cancer: A retrospective cohort study. Surgical Endoscopy. 2013;**27**(1):286-294

[40] Park DJ, Han SU, Hyung WJ, Kim MC, Kim W, Ryu SY, et al. Long-term outcomes after laparoscopy-assisted gastrectomy for advanced gastric cancer: A large-scale multicenter retrospective study. Surgical Endoscopy. 2012;**26**(6):1548-1553

[41] Kitano S, Shiraishi N, Uyama I, Sugihara K, Tanigawa N, Japanese Laparoscopic Surgery Study Group. A multicenter study on oncologic outcome of laparoscopic gastrectomy for early cancer in Japan. Annals of Surgery. 2007;**245**(1):68-72

[42] Kim MC, Kim W, Kim HH, Ryu SW, Ryu SY, Song KY, et al. Risk factors associated with complication following laparoscopy-assisted Gastrectomy for gastric cancer: A large-scale Korean multicenter study. Annals of Surgical Oncology. 2008;**15**(10):2692-2700

3

The Evolution of Minimally Invasive Techniques in Restoration of Colonic Continuity

Stefan H.E.M. Clermonts, Laurents P.S. Stassen and
David D.E. Zimmerman

Abstract

Restoration of bowel continuity after Hartmann's procedure is considered technically challenging and is associated with high morbidity and mortality. This is the main reason why restoration of intestinal continuity is often not attempted. Over the past decade, considerable international experience has gained on this topic with new minimally invasive techniques being developed. This review details the evolution of minimally invasive techniques in restoration of colonic continuity after Hartmann's procedure. A comprehensive search of PubMed and Embase was done. Different restoration modalities were included. Eight studies, from six different countries, in which multiport laparoscopic restoration of continuity was compared to conventional open restoration of bowel continuity, were included. In the total of 254 patients, continuity was restored laparoscopically compared with 255 patients in which continuity was performed in open fashion. Restoration of bowel continuity via trephine access was also reported; three studies including 37 patients were included in this review. Single-port restoration of bowel continuity after Hartmann's procedure is a natural evolution of multiport laparoscopy and trephine access. Six studies reporting on single-port reversal of Hartmann's procedure were included with a total of 75 patients. Single-port access in combination with a transanal approach has also been reported; however, data are extremely limited as there is only one study in the published literature. Success of restoration of bowel continuity with less morbidity and mortality has been demonstrated throughout the evolution of the different surgical techniques. In this review advantages of different approaches for restoration of bowel continuity after Hartmann's procedure are discussed. Furthermore, surgical techniques are described, pictorial guides are added for some techniques, and flowcharts are given for easy use during clinical decision-making.

Keywords: Hartmann's procedure, restoration, intestinal continuity, surgical techniques, laparoscopic, minimal invasive, single-port laparoscopy

1. Introduction

In this chapter we would like to focus on the restoration of intestinal continuity after Hartmann's procedure in general and highlight emerging minimally invasive techniques in specific.

Historically, restoration of bowel continuity after Hartmann's procedure has been considered technically challenging and is associated with high morbidity and mortality rates even despite modern surgical techniques. This is the main reason why restoration of intestinal continuity is often not attempted. Intraoperative difficulties during laparotomy or multiport laparoscopy are mainly caused by the formation of adhesions at the laparotomy site and lower part of the abdomen after active inflammation and/or infection and previous surgery.

The use of the former colostomy site as access to the abdominal cavity has gained some popularity recently. Placing a single-port access system in the former colostomy site combines the potential benefits of minimally invasive surgery (shorter postoperative recovery time, minimal postoperative hospital stay, and lower morbidity rates) with the advantages of Hartmann's reversal through the colostomy site (the absence of new incisions and decreased necessity of midline adhesiolysis).

2. Hartmann's procedure: historical perspective

Henri Albert Hartmann was born on June 16, 1860. Hartmann finished his medical school at the University of Paris on December 19, 1881.

Hartmann starts his internship with Felix Terrier at Hôpital Bichat, who was considered to be one of the most authoritative surgeons at that time [1]. After finishing his surgical training in 1887, Hartmann was appointed as an assistant professor in 1895 and in 1909 as a professor and chairman of the Department of Surgery in 1892. In 1914, Hartman became the chief of Surgery at l'Hôtel-Dieu hospital in Paris (**Figure 1**) [2]. During his lengthy and extraordinary career, Hartmann meticulously recorded each operation he performed. Upon his retirement he had documented around 30,000 cases [3].

Hartmann's procedure was first described in 1921 [4, 5]. In his first patients with obstructive carcinoma of the sigmoid, he performed a proximal colostomy and then a sigmoid resection with closure of the rectal stump via an abdominal approach. He developed this technique in response to high mortality rates in his patients who underwent an abdominoperineal resection, as first described by Miles in 1908 [1]. In 1931 Hartmann described the procedure in detail in his book *Chirurgie du Rectum* (**Figure 2**).

Although Hartmann developed his technique mainly for rectal cancer, in present times, Hartmann's procedure is often the preferred procedure for severe diverticulitis of the sigmoid. Despite Hartmann never intended restoration of bowel continuity, recent publications showed that a direct reconstruction is feasible in selected patients [6].

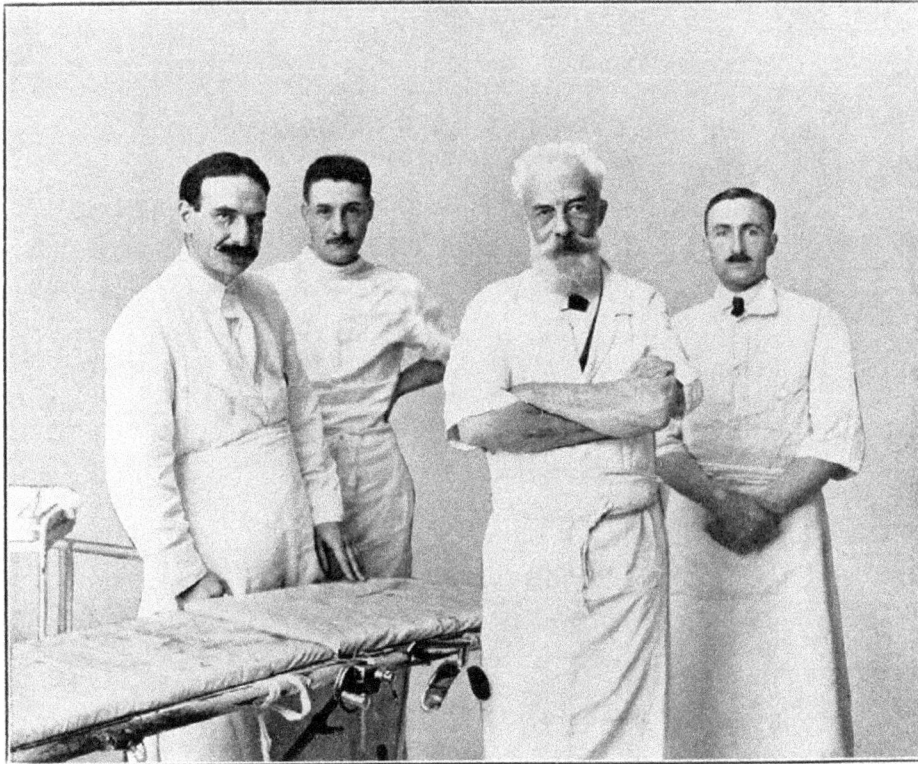

Figure 1. Henri Hartmann (second from the right) and his three assistants, Drs. Bergeret, Gouverneur, and Huet, at the Hotel-Dieu, Paris. Source image: http://wellcomeimages.org.

2.1. Reversal of Hartmann's procedure

Hartmann never attempted to reanastomose the bowel in his patients. He believed this would result in unnecessarily high morbidity and mortality [3].

Restoring intestinal continuity after Hartmann's operation is a difficult operation that is associated with a high morbidity rate, with anastomotic leakage rates ranging from 4% to 16% and an operative mortality reported as high as 10% [7–10].

The high incidence of morbidity and mortality is the main reasons why surgeons are reluctant to restore intestinal continuity in approximately 40% of the patients undergoing Hartmann's procedure [10, 11].

2.2. Indications and contraindications

The primary indication for reversal of Hartmann's procedure is curing people of the discomforts that are caused by the end colostomy. Patients with stomas face many physical and psychological challenges, including leakage, skin rashes, lifestyle alterations, and sexual dysfunction [12, 13].

Literature defines no contraindications for reversal of Hartmann's procedure. However, a review of the literature covering restoration after Hartmann's procedure shows that advanced age, ASA grade 3, or higher and fecal peritonitis at the time of Hartmann's procedure are

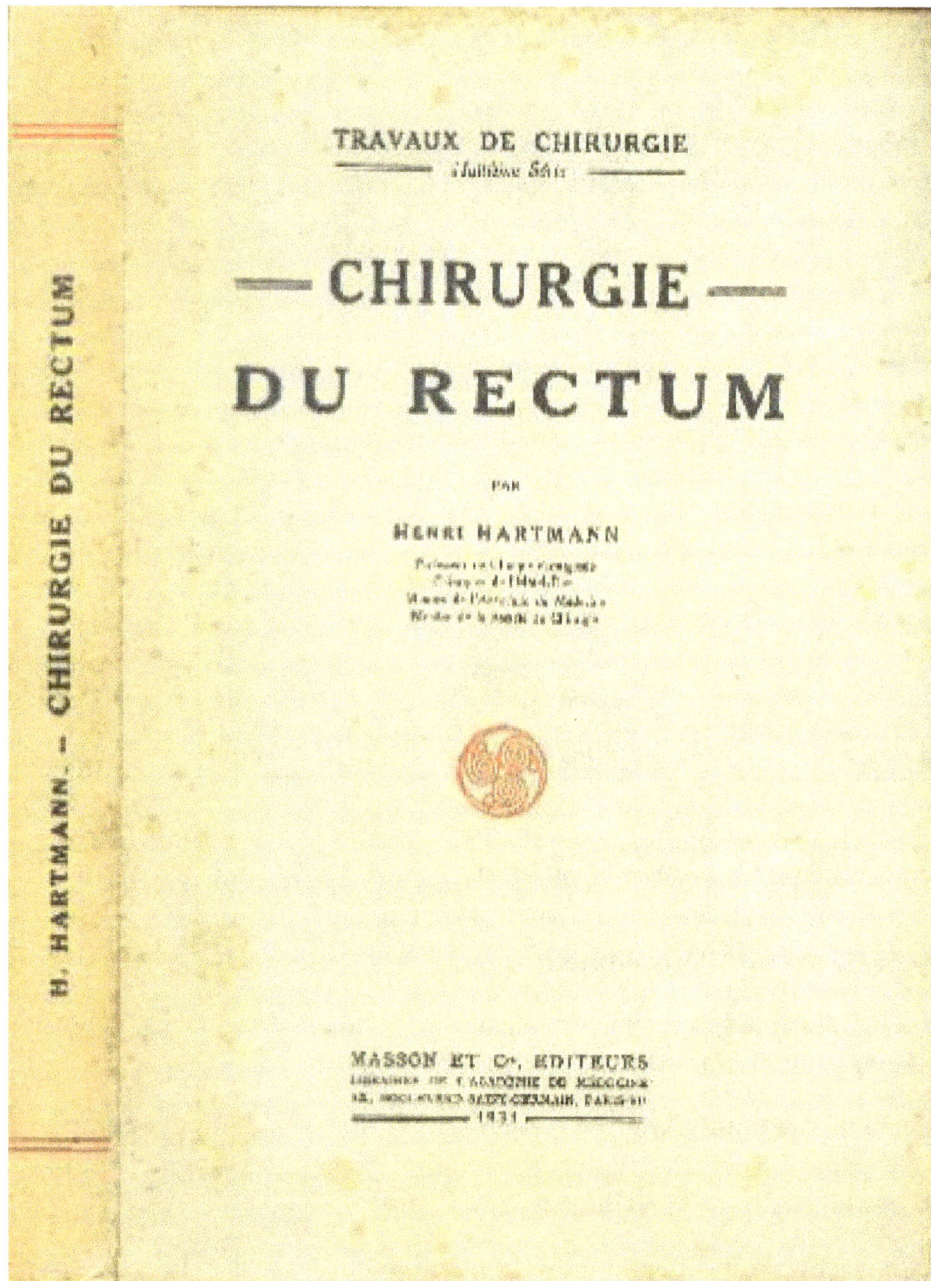

Figure 2. Cover of the book *Chirurgie du rectum* by Henri Hartmann. Published 1931. Source image: http://archive.org.

often considered relevant contraindications. Roque-Castellano and colleagues analyzed factors related to the decision of restoring intestinal continuity. They found that female sex and neoplastic disorders are relative contraindications for restoration of intestinal continuity [14]. Furthermore, we believe there must be some reluctance to perform conventional restoration of bowel continuity by laparotomy in patients with an incisional hernia. The reason for this statement is the need for repair of the incisional hernia and the restoration of the bowel continuity at the same time. This reluctance is following the dictum that abdominal wall prostheses must be avoided during contaminated operations [15]. The authors advocate the use of single-port laparoscopic reversal of Hartmann's procedure in case of an incisional hernia. With this modality the midline can be left unchanged rendering concomitant repair of the incisional hernia unnecessary. The single-port laparoscopic technique will be discussed in detail in Section 5.1.

2.3. Preoperative workup

Prior to the restoration of the intestinal continuity, routine evaluation of the rectal stump and descending colon is often performed in order to detect stump leakage, cavity formation, or strictures and establish the length of the rectal stump. The integrity and patency of the rectal stump are evaluated by physical examination, flexible endoscopy and/or radiographically by contrast proctography CT scan. Despite these routine practices, little data exist to support this in case of restoration of bowel continuity after Hartmann's procedure. Data do exist on the routine use of contrast enema prior to the closure of a defunctioning ileostomy in patients with low pelvic anastomosis is inconsistent when its sole purpose is detecting leaks or cavity formation [16–18]. These studies show that strictures or narrowing of the bowel lumen is seldom detected. In cases where strictures are detected, dilatation is performed without the need for cancelation the reversal of the – ostomy. When extrapolating these findings, it is questionable whether routine contrast studies are necessary in the case of Hartmann's reversal. Moreover, usually patients who develop an anastomotic leak of the rectal stump present with clinical symptoms long before restoration of the bowel continuity is scheduled. However, in patients where initial Hartmann's procedure was acutely performed for neoplastic disorders, direct visualization of the rectal stump and remaining colon is mandatory to exclude recurrence of the malignancy or other neoplastic lesions. Based on these limited data, the authors advocate performing flexible rectoscopy to ensure viability of the rectal stump and the absence of remaining diverticular disease or local recurrence in case of prior malignancy. Data on routinely performing X-ray or contrast enema is limited to expert opinions and therefore not mandatory. Authors' recommendations are summarized in the algorithm in **Figure 3**.

2.4. Timing of surgery

There is limited data available concerning the optimal timing of restoration of continuity. Most surgeons will postpone surgery for at least 6 months after the initial operation, obviously depending on the current health and recuperation of the patient. It has been suggested by Keck and coworkers that a waiting period of 15 weeks may be beneficial [19]. It is however noteworthy that reversing Hartmann's procedure after a shorter period did not influence morbidity or mortality, but did seem to lengthen the duration of hospitalisation and increase the perceived operative difficulty (and thus the risk). Other authors have also suggested there is no indication to delay closure for longer than 16 weeks [20]. Based on these limited data, the authors advocate a minimal waiting period of 4 months between the initial operation and restoration of continuity in order to maximize the possibility of minimally invasive techniques for restoring continuity.

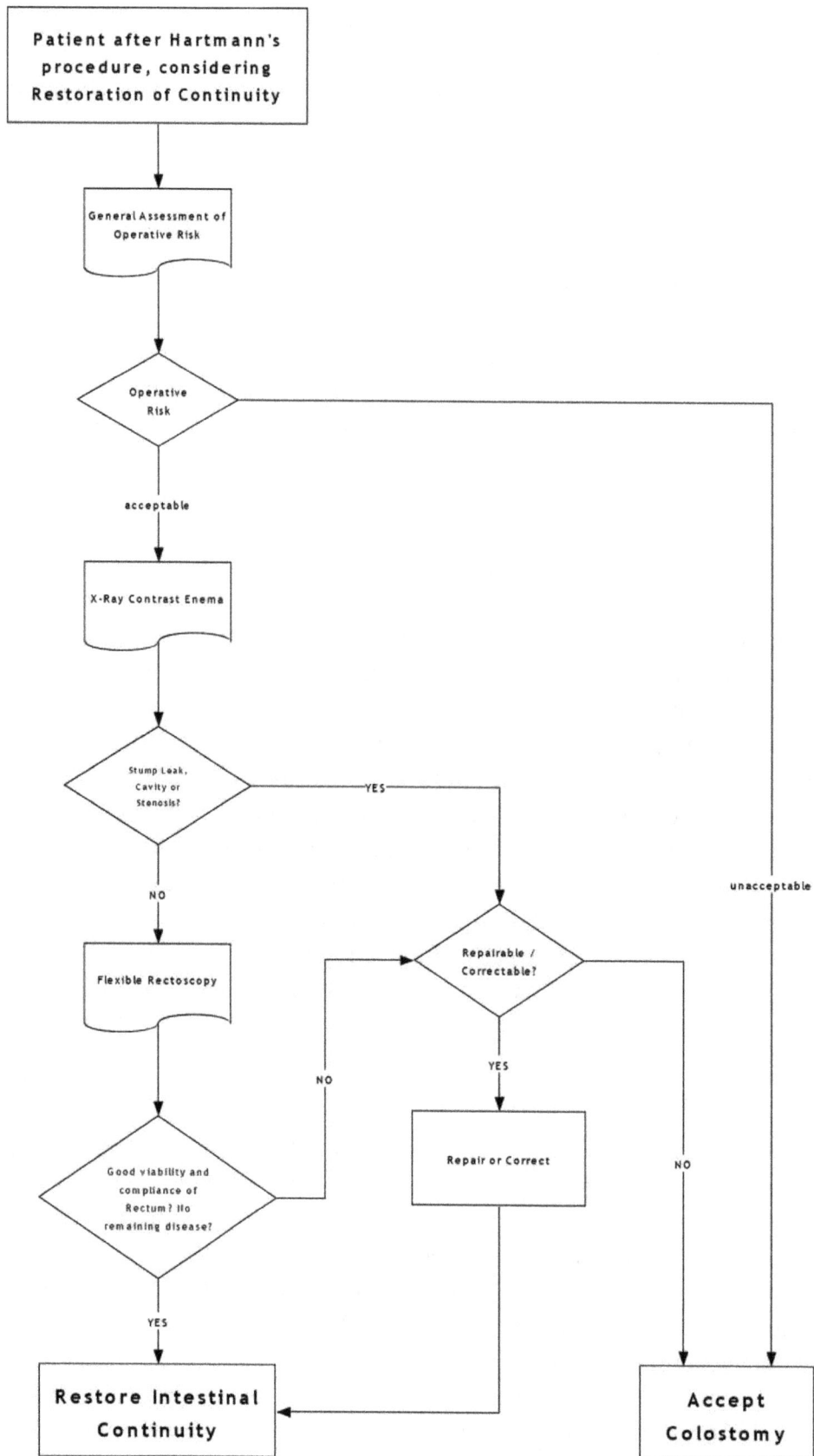

Figure 3. Algorithm advocated to be used during decision-making and the preoperative workup for restoration of bowel continuity after Hartmann's procedure.

3. Surgical techniques for restoration of intestinal continuity after Hartmann's procedure

Reestablishing bowel continuity after Hartmann's procedure is considered a major surgical procedure that is accompanied by considerable morbidity and mortality. Multiport laparoscopy was the first technique in a sequence of attempts to reduce the high morbidity and mortality that is associated with this procedure.

3.1. Multiport laparoscopic reversal of Hartmann's procedure

The patient is placed in a supine position. Next, there are two different ways to continue the procedure. In one option the procedure is initiated with mobilization of the stoma to the level of the abdominal wall and then freeing the ostomy from the fascia. The alternative procedure starts by insertion of a 10 mm camera trocar and a working trocar when needed (**Figure 4**), establishing the pneumoperitoneum, and perform a prior inspection for factors that could potentially cause abortion later on in the procedure. We advocate starting the procedure in the latter fashion, since this technique facilitates early decision-making by the surgeon on continuing or aborting the procedure when a potential unsuccessful bowel restoration is anticipated. Consequently, there is no need for refashioning of the end colostomy.

In both techniques the next step is transecting the colon using a linear stapler to remove the end of the colostomy and securing the anvil of a circular stapler is secured with a purse-string suture, in the proximal colon. The descending colon is then returned into the abdominal cavity. Any adhesions in the abdominal cavity are freed to enable insertion of the other ports. The colostomy site is closed using a wound protector/retractor device with a laparoscopic cap so that it can function as an additional working port. The pneumoperitoneum is then established. Additional 5 mm working trocars are placed in the right upper quadrant and right iliac fossa. Extensive dissection of adhesions from the anterior abdominal wall in the midline is mandatory with this multi-port technique in order to cross the midline (**Figure 4**).

The small bowel is mobilized from the left iliac fossa and out of the pelvis. The proximal descending colon would have been mobilized to a varying extent at the initial Hartmann's procedure, and this will need to be redone, including the splenic flexure. A rectal probe or circular stapler sizer is used to identify the rectal stump. In order to perform an end-to-end anastomosis, further mobilization and adhesiolysis of the rectal stump are sometimes necessary. Alternatively, if mobilization is difficult and the anterior rectal wall can clearly be identified and adequate length of the descending colon is available to allow a tension-free anastomosis, an side-to-side anastomosis can be performed. A circular stapler is introduced into the rectum to fashion the anastomosis. The stapler is deployed and the donuts are checked. Next, we advocate performing an additional leak test as this is associated with reduced rates of postoperative adverse events in literature [21]. The pneumoperitoneum is released, and the trocars are removed under direct visualization. The fascia is then closed in apertures equal to or larger than 10 mm.

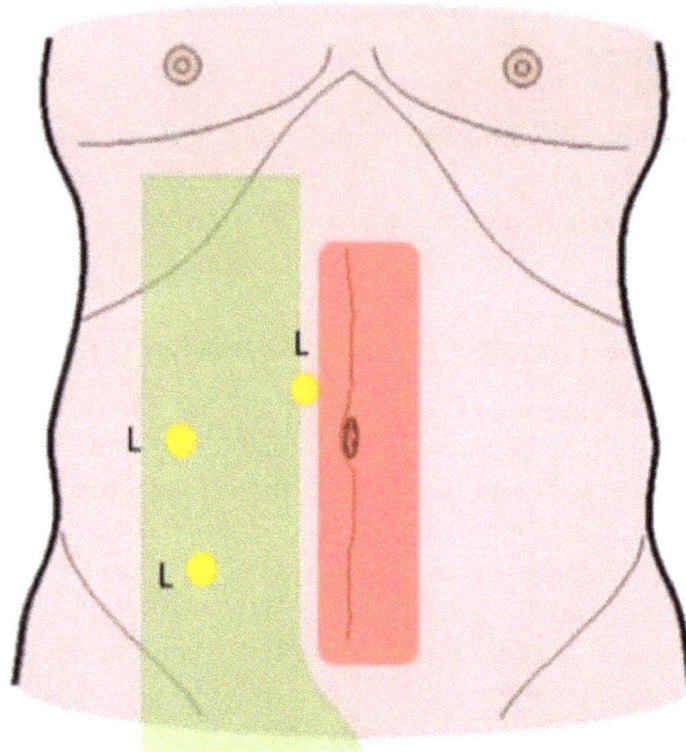

Figure 4. Port positions for multiport laparoscopic Hartmann's reversal. L = laparoscopic trocar position. *Red-shaded area*: area of maximal adhesion formation after previous laparotomy. *Green-shaded area*: area of range of action that is relatively free of adhesions. Note that in this technique the midline has to be crossed.

3.2. The open technique compared to multiport laparoscopic restoration technique: an appraisal of the literature

In recent literature a limited amount of studies compared an open approach with the multiport laparoscopic technique [22–31]. In **Table 1** a summary of studies on multiport laparoscopic versus conventional Hartmann's reversal is presented.

As expected, for the minimal invasive technique, the total length of hospital stay was shorter with 6.9 days when compared to the open approach that shows a mean of 10.4 days. Furthermore, for patients in whom bowel continuity was restored laparoscopically, overall morbidity rates seemed lower when compared to patients who were treated conventionally. In the laparoscopic group, mean morbidity rates were 12% versus 20% in the open group. The main and foremost complications after bowel restoration for both modalities are summarized in **Table 2**.

In the reviewed literature, mortality seems comparable for both techniques, with a mean mortality of 0.9% in the laparoscopic group and 1.2% in the conventional group. No statistically significant differences were found for mean total operation time, 150 minutes for the laparoscopic technique and 172 minutes for conventional procedures. A possible explanation for the relative long operation duration for both techniques is the extensive adhesiolysis that is required. 80 percent of the conversions from laparoscopy to the conventional technique arises for this reason [33], resulting in an average conversion rate of 12 percent. In the opinion of the authors, there is no place for primary open restoration of continuity after Hartmann's

Study	Country	Year of publication	Procedure	Number of patients	Morbidity (%)	Mortality (%)	Operation time (mean min)	Hospital stay (days)	Control group (number of patients)	Morbidity (%)	Mortality (%)	Operation time (mean min)	Hospital stay (days)
Rosen et al. [24]	USA	2005	Laparoscopic	20	3 (14)	0 (0)	158	4.2	No				NS
Faure et al. [25]	FR	2007	Laparoscopic	14	2 (14.2)	0 (0)	143	9.5	Conventional (20)	6 (30)	0 (0)	180	11
Haughn et al. [26]	USA	2008	Laparoscopic	61	8 (13)	0 (0)	154	NS	Conventional (61)	11 (18)	0(0)	210	NS
Vermeulen et al. [27]	NL	2008	Laparoscopic	3	(15.8)*	(5)*	NS	NS	Conventional(48)	(15.8)*	(5)*	NS	NS
Mazeh et al. [28]	IL	2009	Laparoscopic	82	15 (17.6)	0 (0)	193	6.5	Conventional (41)	15 (36.5)	0 (0)	209	8.1
Di Carlo et al. [29]	IT	2010	Laparoscopic	3	0 (0)	0 (0)	95.6	NS	Conventional (3)	0 (0)	0 (0)	136.6	NS
De'angelis et al. [30]	FR	2013	Laparoscopic	28	3 (10.7)	0 (0)	171.1	6.7	Conventional (18)	6 (33.6)	0 (0)	235.8	11.2
Yang et al. [31]	AU	2014	Laparoscopic	43	6 (14)	0 (0)	276.4	6.7	Conventional (64)	20 (31)	0 (0)	242	10.8

AU, Australia; FR, France; IT, Italy; IL, Israel; NL, the Netherlands; USA, United States of America; NS, not stated. In the study by Vermeulen et al. [32]. Subdivision is made for laparoscopic or conventional reversal; therefore, only overall morbidity and mortality are given for this study.

Table 1. Summary of current literature that compares multiport laparoscopic Hartmann's reversal versus the conventional open technique.

	Type of intestinal continuity restoration	
	Multiport laparoscopy	Laparotomy
Hemorrhage	1.7	3
Wound infection	10.6	14
Anastomotic leakage	1.2	5
Reoperation	4	7
Cardiopulmonary	3.6	7

Values are derived from the literature. Values are in mean percentages.

Table 2. Morbidity rates depicted for multiport laparoscopic reversal of Hartmann's procedure compared with conventional reversal.

procedure, due to unnecessary morbidity, mortality, and trauma to the abdominal wall. We advocate selection of a minimally invasive procedure.

4. Trephine access: using the former colostomy site as access point

Although laparoscopic restoration of the intestinal continuity has many advantages, in laparoscopic reversal of Hartmann's procedure, an extended adhesiolysis in the midline and pelvis is still needed. This adhesiolysis may increase postoperative paralytic ileus and the risk of inadvertent bowel lacerations.

The use of the colostomy site as an even less invasive method for access to the abdominal cavity and restoration of the intestinal continuity was first described by Vermeulen and colleagues in 2008 [32]. In this technique manual access is gained through the stoma site in combination with a blindly performed adhesiolysis without laparoscopic assistance (**Figure 5**). This procedure was called the SIR method "stoma incision reversal" procedure.

4.1. SIR procedure: surgical technique

The patient is positioned in the lithotomy. The stoma is released, taking a small amount of surrounding skin with it. Then the colostomy is closed provisionally with a running suture. The length of the incision at the stomal site must be large enough to fit the surgeon's hand. The descending colon stump is brought outside the abdomen; visible adhesions connected to the left colon are sharply dissected. Further adhesiolysis of the left colon is performed manually between the thumb and index finger in order to create enough length for the descending colon to reach the pelvic cavity. If enough bowel length is created. The anvil of a circular stapler is placed intraluminal. The stump is closed using a linear stapler. The tip of the stapler anvil is brought through the colon the staple line and tied by a purse-string suture. The descending colon with the anvil is returned intra-abdominally. For the next step, the surgeon's right hand is placed intra-abdominally through the former colostomy side. The left hand is used to transanally introduce a rigid sizer to identify and manipulate the rectal stump. Adhesions between the rectal stump and adjacent small bowels are loosened manually and blindly with the surgeon's right hand. Consecutively, the circular stapler is introduced into

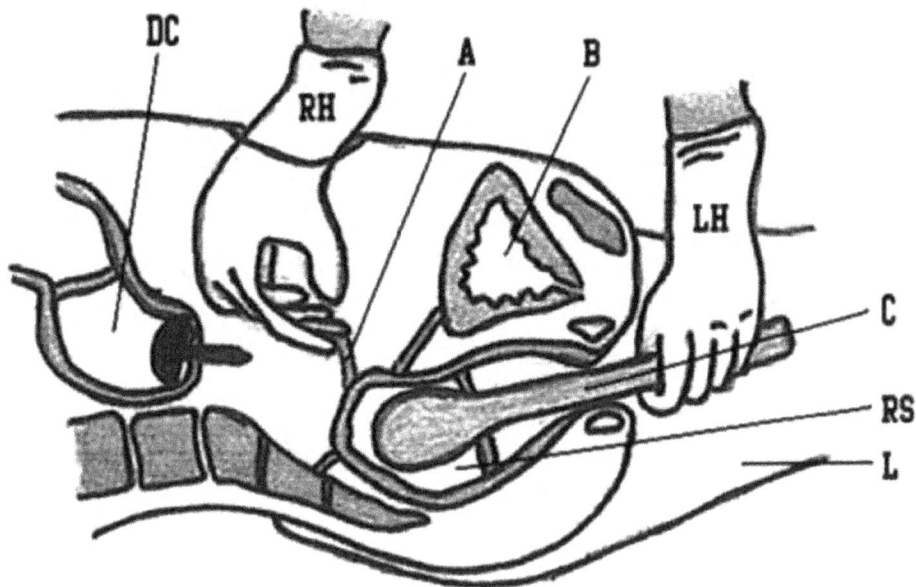

Figure 5. Manual lysis of adhesions at the tip of the rectal stump, which was identified using a rigid club. Previously, the anvil of a circular stapler was placed intraluminal of the descending colon. DC, descending colon with anvil; RH, right hand; A, adhesions; B, bladder; LH, left hand; C, rigid club; RS, rectal stump; L, left leg. Source: Ref. [34].

the rectal stump. The pin of the circular stapler is passed through the rectal wall, and the anvil is attached. Before firing the circular stapler, the proximal bowel segment is manually checked for rotation and interposition. After firing the stapler, the integrity of the doughnuts of the anastomosis is inspected, and a leak test is performed. The fascia is closed with a PDS suture, and the skin as deemed appropriate.

4.2. Appraisal of the literature

A review of the literature shows three studies [32, 34–36] on the SIR technique. **Table 3** summarizes the results. Vermeulen and colleagues described the first pilot study in 2010. They attempted the procedure in 13 consecutive patients with a median age of 56 years (range 35–81 years). Indications for initial surgery were iatrogenic bowel perforation ($n = 3$), intestinal bowel obstruction due to complicated diverticulitis ($n = 3$), and diverticulitis ($n = 7$). Median delay of reversal was 7 months.

Of the 13 patients assigned for reversal of Hartmann's procedure through the stomal site, two patients needed direct conversion to laparotomy due to firm adhesions. Of the 11 patients in which the procedure was accomplished through the stoma site, mean operation time was 81 min (range 58–109 min) with a mean hospital stay of 4.2 days. No anastomotic leaks occurred. In 2010 Vermeulen and colleagues published the results of their "stoma incision reversal" procedure in 22 patients and compare the results with matched cases in which restoration of the intestinal continuity was performed by laparotomy. In the "SIR" group, five procedures were converted to laparotomy due to firm adhesions ($n = 2$), doubt about the quality of the doughnuts ($n = 2$), or iatrogenic small bowel lacerations ($n = 1$).

In this study the mean operation time was significantly shorter when performing the SIR procedure (75 min (58–208)) compared to the open group (141 min (85–276)) ($p < 0.001$). Patients

Study	Country	Year of publication	Number of patients	Procedure	Control group (number of patients)	Morbidity (%)	Mortality (%)	Operation time (mean min)	Hospital stay (days)
Vermeulen et al. [32]	NL	2008	13	Trephine access	No (0)	0 (0)	0 (0)	81	4.2
Vermeulen et al. [34]	NL	2010	16	Trephine access	Yes (32)	4 (25)	0 (0)	75	4
Aydin et al. [35]	TR	2011	8	Trephine access	No (0)	0 (0)	0	65	5.5

NL, the Netherlands; TR, Turkey.

Table 3. Summary of "trephine access" technique reversal of Hartmann's procedure in the current literature.

	Type of intestinal continuity restoration	
	"SIR"	Laparotomy
Total complications	4	16
Anastomotic leakage	1	2
Ileus	0	1
Wound infections	1	5
Urine retention	1	0
Incisional hernia	1	8
Mortality	0	1
Vermeulen et al. 2010 [35].		

Table 4. Postoperative complications after restoration of bowel continuity depicted for the "SIR" procedure (trephine access) and conventional technique.

who underwent the SIR procedure had a shorter postoperative hospital stay (SIR group range 2-7 days) ($p < 0.001$). The total postoperative number of complications was not significantly different between both procedures. Twenty-five percent for the SIR patients versus 50% of the patients that were treated by the conventional technique. Postoperative complications after bowel continuity restoration are depicted in **Table 4**.

In 2011 Aydin and colleagues perform the aforementioned technique in eight patients. Indications for the initial Hartmann's procedure were sigmoid volvulus ($n = 4$), obstructive sigmoid cancer ($n = 2$), rectal trauma ($n = 2$), and Fournier's gangrene ($n = 1$). The mean duration between the primary procedure and reversal of the Hartmann's procedure was 5 months (range 2–8 months). All patients included had a body mass index of less than 30 km/m^2 and a rectal stump of at least 5 cm. In two patients the incision was extended from the stoma site for better visualization of the rectal stump in one patient and due to injury of the intestine in one patient. Mean duration of the operation was 65 min (range 45–80 min). No postoperative complications were observed. Patients were discharged after a mean of 5.5 days (range 4–9 days). Aydin and coworkers note that this technique should ideally be used in non-obese patients with long rectal stumps of sufficient length.

The SIR technique originated in the Netherlands and met criticism due to the blind nature of the dissection phase of the procedure. Regarding the risk of blind dissection as well as the availability of improved access platforms that enable adequate vision and control, the authors do not advocate the use of the SIR technique in present times.

5. Single-port restoration of the intestinal continuity through the stoma trephine site

Single-port restoration of intestinal continuity with access through the formal site of the colostomy is a relatively new technique. The main goal for the development of this method is introducing a minimally invasive technique that further reduces the morbidity and mortality of a procedure that is technically demanding and complex.

5.1. Surgical technique

The patient is placed in lithotomy position. Primarily, the colostomy is mobilized and freed from the fascia (**Figure 6**). The mobilized descending colon is then pulled out of the abdomen and exposed (**Figure 7**). Next, the colon is transected using a linear stapler to remove the end colostomy, and the anvil of a circular stapler is secured with a purse-string suture, in the proximal colon. Either a terminal or lateral position can be chosen (**Figure 8**). The descending colon is returned into the abdominal cavity. Any adhesions close to the wound in the abdominal cavity on direct view are freed. The single-port access platform is then placed in the fascial defect at the colostomy site, and the pneumoperitoneum is then established (**Figure 9**). A rigid 30-degree laparoscope is introduced and a diagnostic laparoscopy is performed. Subsequently, the patient

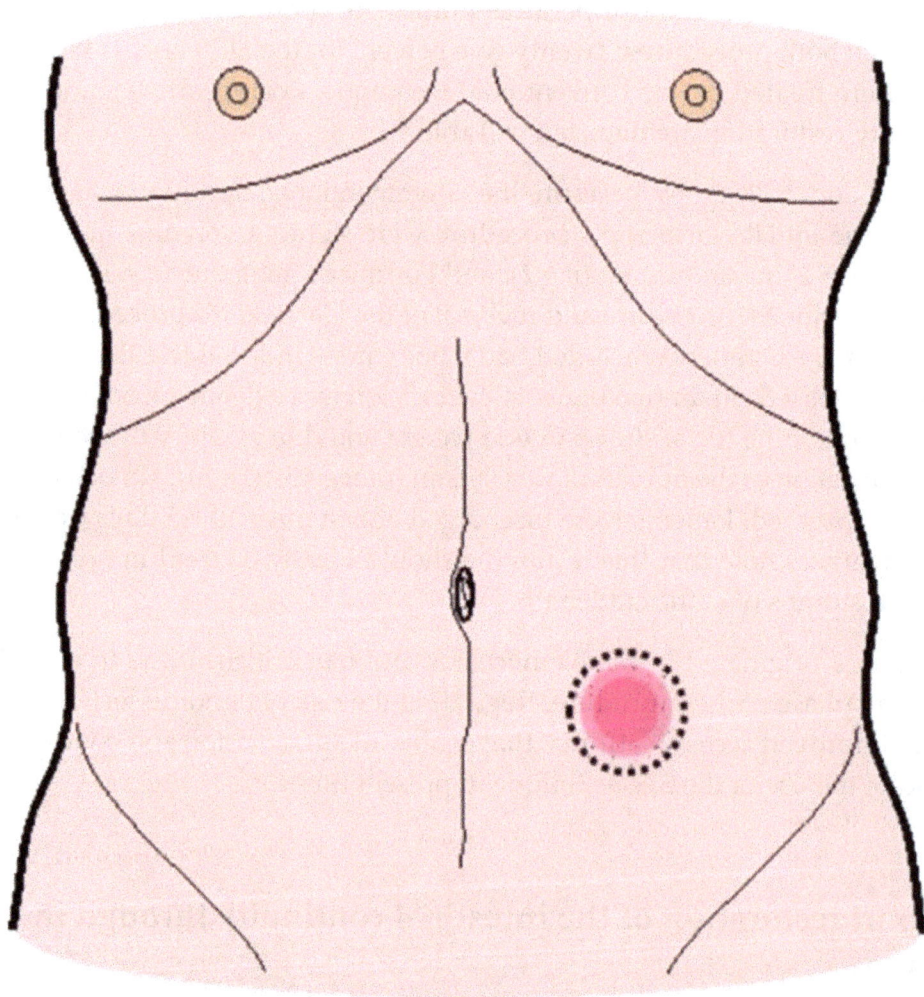

Figure 6. Release of the colostomy.

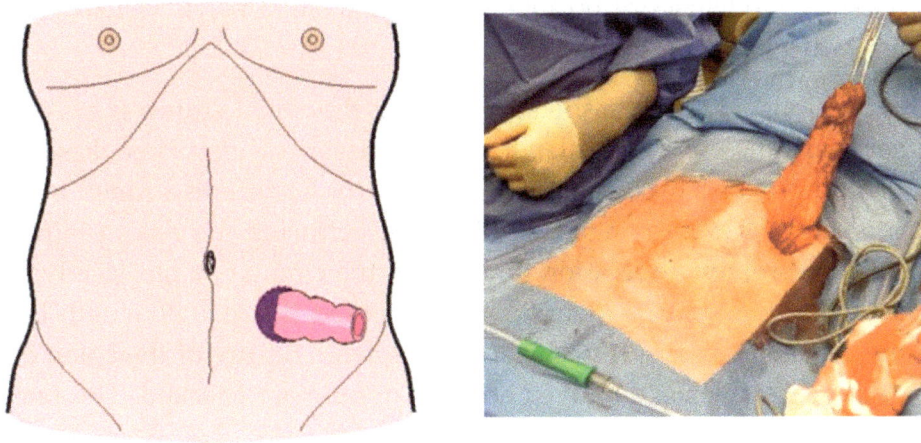

Figure 7. Mobilization of the descending colon with sufficient length.

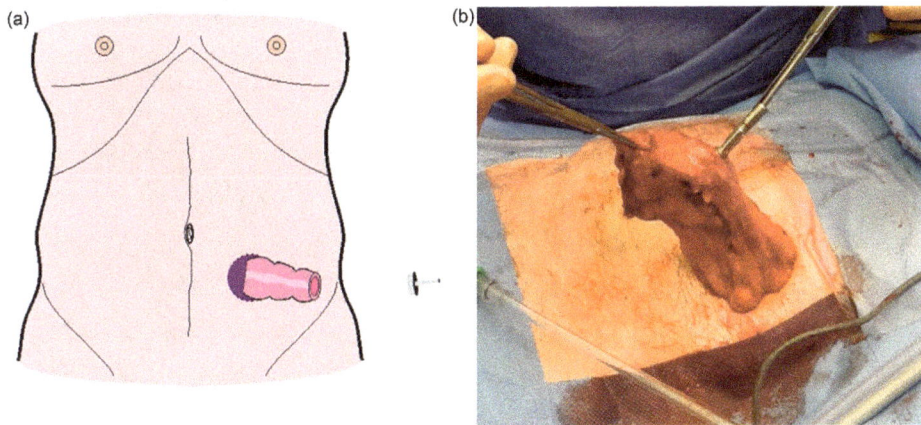

Figure 8. Insertion of the anvil of the circular stapler. Left picture shows a terminal position. Right picture shows a lateral positioning of the anvil for side-to-end configuration.

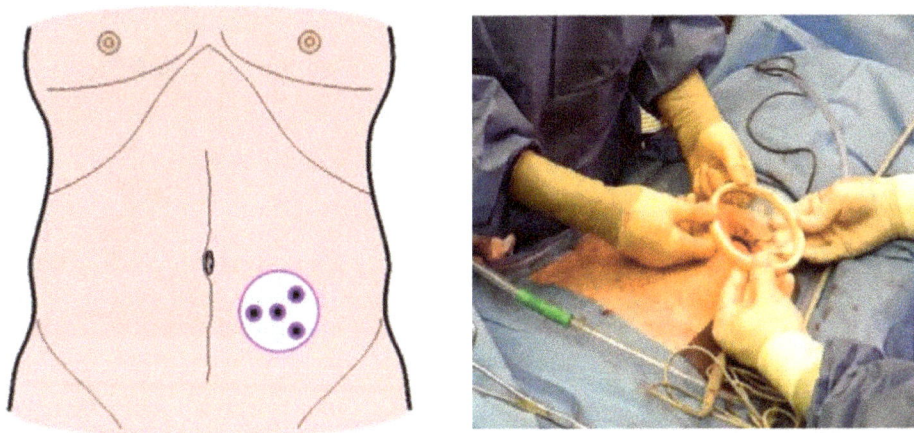

Figure 9. Placement of the single-port access device in the fascia defect at the formal stoma site. Right picture shows the placement of the flexible wound protector.

is positioned in anti-Trendelenburg position making the small pelvis visible. Adhesiolysis is performed using two 5 mm working trocars.

Dissection of adhesions and scar tissue surrounding the rectal stump is performed extensively, by either sharp dissection with laparoscopic scissors or ultrasonic dissection devices, until the rectal stump is as bare as possible (**Figure 10**). Adhesions formed at the previous midline incision can be left unchanged at this stage, reducing the risk of iatrogenic bowel perforation and reducing total operation time. Next, the circular stapler is advanced via the anus, and the descending colon is identified and checked if adequate length is available to allow a tension-free anastomosis. If necessary, the splenic flexure of the colon can be mobilized (**Figure 11**). The stapler is deployed and the donuts are checked. The pneumoperito-

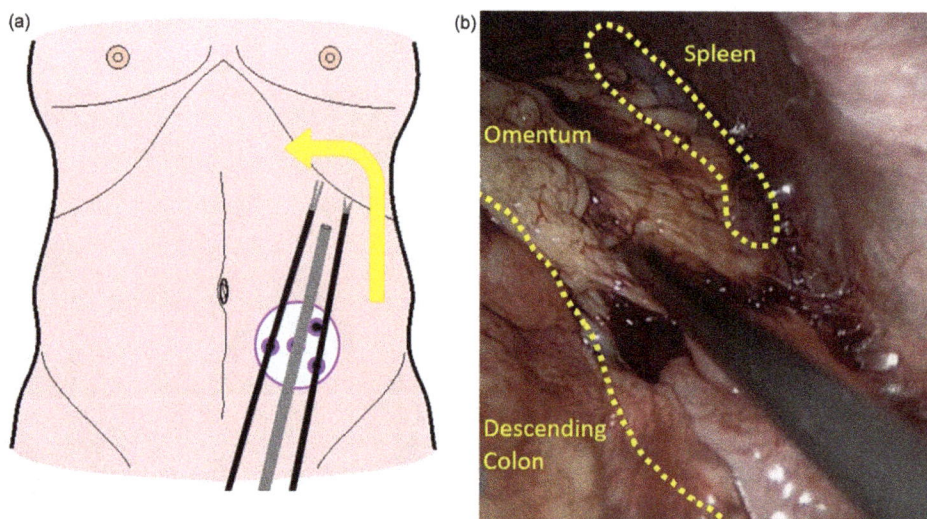

Figure 10. Adhesiolysis and mobilization of the splenic flexure.

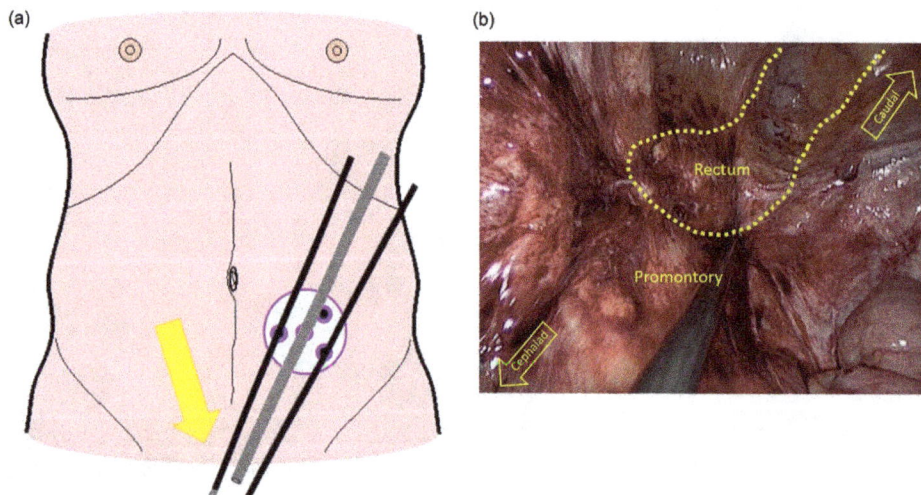

Figure 11. Dissection of adhesions and scar tissue surrounding the rectal stump.

Study	Country	Year of publication	Number of patients	Procedure	Control group (number of patients)	Morbidity (%)	Mortality (%)	Hospital stay(days)
Smith et al. [42]	USA	2011	1	Stoma site. Single port	No (0)	0(0)	0(0)	5
Carus et al. [39]	GE	2011	8	Stoma site. Single port	No (0)	1 (12.5)	0 (0)	4
Borowski et al. [38]	UK	2011	5	Stoma site. Single port	No (0)	1 (20)	0	4.2
Joshi et al. [41]	UK	2013	14	Stoma site. Glove port	No (0)	3 (21)	0 (0)	5.5
Choi et al. [40]	KR	2015	22	Stoma site. Glove port. Single port	No (0)	4 (18.2)	0(0)	8
Clermonts et al. [37]	NL	2016	25	Stoma site. Single port	Yes (16)	8 (32)	0 (0)	4

KR, Korea; NL, the Netherlands; UK, the United Kingdom; GE, Germany; USA, the United States of America.

Table 5. Summary of single-port reversal of Hartmann's procedure in the current literature.

neum is released and the trocars are removed under direct visualization. The fascia is then closed in apertures equal to or larger than 10 mm.

5.2. Appraisal of the literature

A review of the literature reveals that only a few small case series have been published on this technique. At the moment no randomized controlled trials were published [37–42]. **Table 5** summarizes the results of the available literature. The technique was first described by Smith and colleagues [42]; in this case single-port restoration of the intestinal continuity was performed in a 56-year-old patient with a history of perforated diverticulosis. Their total operation time was 104 min. The patient started a clear liquid diet on postoperative day 2 and was discharged after 5 days. The largest study without control patients was that of Choi et al. [40] and consisted of 23 patients. In one patient closure of the colostomy was aborted due to intraoperative difficulties. The median age of their patients was 62 years (range 21–87 years), with an overall ASA grade of II. Median time to reversal was 153.5 days (range 99–1028). Main indications for Hartmann's procedure were: complicated diverticulitis (27.3%), colorectal carcinoma (27.3%), and sigmoid volvulus (18.2%). They reported a median operation time of 165 minutes (range 100-340 minutes) and a total hospital stay of 8 days (range 4–31 days). There morbidity rate was 18.2% with two reoperations, one for anastomotic dehiscence and one for rectovesical fistula. No mortality was reported. Carus and colleagues' study consisted of 8 patients with a median age of 60.4 years (range 36–84). Hartmann's procedure was performed for complicated diverticulitis (five laparoscopic, three open). The reversal was performed 2–4 months after the primary procedure. No conversions were reported in one procedure; they had to play one extra trocar had to be placed during adhesiolysis; and one patient with a superficial wound infection (morbidity 12.5%). No mortality was reported. Patients were discharged after a median of 6.4 days (range 4–8 days). The series by Clermonts et al. [37] was the only study that included a control group. They included a total of 25 patients (median age, 52.2 years). Indications for primary surgery consisted of complicated diverticulitis (60%) and malignancy in 28% of the cases. Median time to reversal was 16 months. These patients were compared with a control group in which closure of the colostomy was performed in an open method. In the open group, all primary Hartmann's procedures were performed by laparotomy; in the single-port group, 88% was performed by laparotomy. No statistical significant differences were observed between the two groups. Median operation time in the single-port group

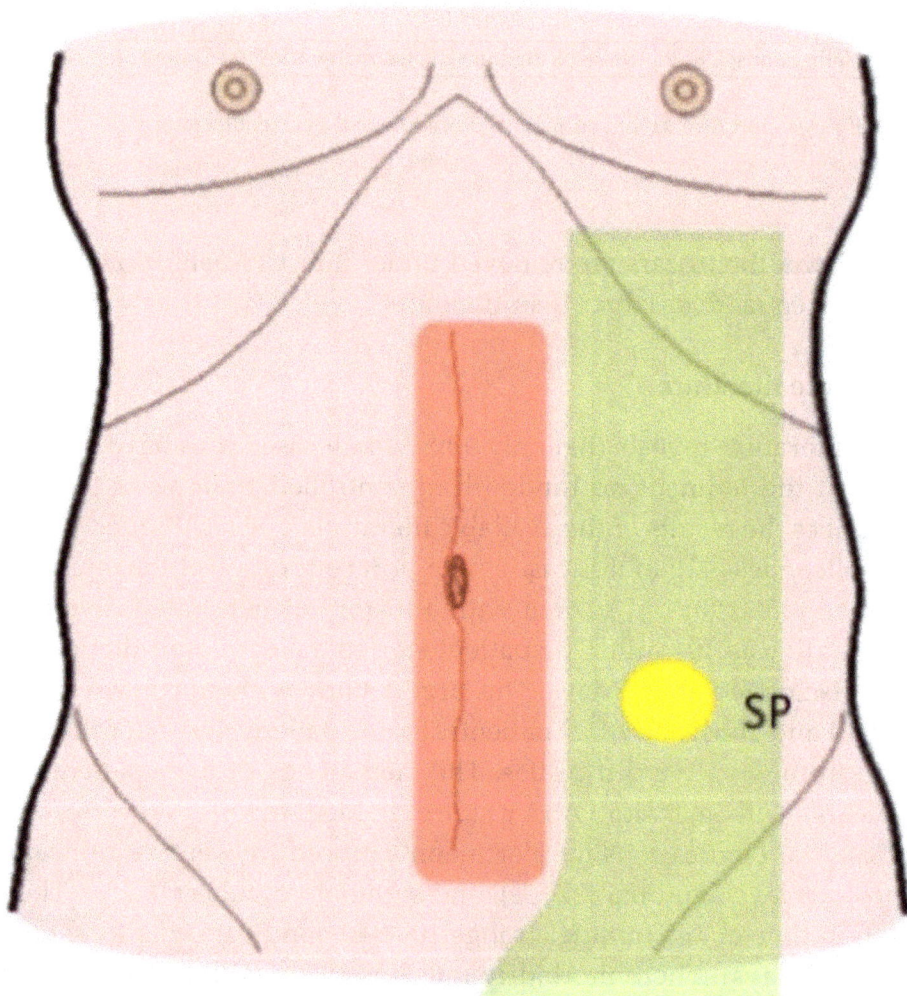

Figure 12. Port position for single-port Hartmann's reversal. SP = single-port trocar position. *Red-shaded area*: area of maximal adhesion formation after previous laparotomy. *Green-shaded area*: area of range of action that is relatively free of adhesions.

was 153.5 min (range: 73–332 minutes) and 184.4 min (range 29–377 minutes) in the open group. One single-port procedure was converted to laparotomy and two procedures to multiport laparoscopy due to difficulties during the adhesiolysis. In the single-port group, a total of eight complications were observed compared with 33 complications in the open group. Wound infections, 5 (20 %) versus 12 (75 %), accounted for the largest number of complications in the SPHR and OHR groups. One patient died after anastomotic leakage and sepsis in the control group; no mortality was observed in the single-port group. The median hospital stay was 4 days in the single-port group compared to a mean of 16 days in the open group.

5.3. Advantages of this technique

Single port restoration of the intestinal continuity has some major advantages over the previously mentioned techniques. The minimally invasive technique has the usual advantages of this technique with less pain and faster recovery. Specifically, in Hartmann's reversal also a shorter operation time is observed. The single port variant using the formal stoma site as an access point has the additional advantage that crossing the midline is avoided, rendering an extensive adhesiolysis unnecessary as **Figure 12** schematically shows.

Another big advantage of minimalizing the access trauma is shown in the very short hospital stay compared to the open and laparoscopic techniques. The small incision, almost no blood loss, and short operation time could be the main reasons.

6. Single-port trephine access and transanal access combined for restoration of the intestinal continuity

In Section 5 we already described the advantages of single-port restoration of intestinal continuity with access through the formal site of the colostomy. Recently, a new technique that combines the single-port trephine access with single-port transanal access was presented [43]. It is suggested the transanal approach will aid in the technically challenging dissection of the rectal stump and perform a pelvic adhesiolysis in a safer manner.

6.1. Surgical technique

Patients receive mechanical bowel and rectal stump cleansing. Patients are placed in lithotomy position. The procedure is performed by two surgeons starting simultaneously; one surgeon starts the abdominal trephine access approach (Section 5). The second surgeon places a single-port transanal access platform through the anal canal with three working trocars. The pneumorectum is created. Next, circular dissection next to the stapler line in the proximal part of the rectal stump is performed into the avascular presacral plane posteriorly. This plane of dissection is extended medially, laterally, and interiorly to achieve the desired circumferential rectal mobilization. Finally, the peritoneal reflection was visualized and divided to achieve the proximal rectal stump removal, with both surgeons working together. The previous stapler line with the resected tissue can be extracted transanally. Next, a Prolene purse-string suture is used to close the distal rectal stump. In order to complete the end-to-end anastomosis, a circular stapler is inserted via the anal canal and connected to the anvil in the proximal descending colon. After firing the circular stapler and completing the anastomosis, the integrity of the anastomosis can be evaluated with an air test, as well as an intraluminal examination through the transanal access platform.

6.2. Critical appraisal of literature

A review of the literature reveals one study by Bravo and colleagues [43]. The study group describes a technique that is easily adopted and mastered by surgeons already trained in transanal colorectal surgery. They report no postoperative morbidity and a quick recovery and discharge from the hospital (no exact numbers given). Furthermore, a shorter total operation time is mentioned when compared to a multiport laparoscopic approach.

Advantages of this technique mentioned by the authors are first of all the safe dissection of the rectal stump because most of the work is done in a surgical plane not touched during the initial surgery and thus without adhesions. This gives the ability to precisely identify structures with adherence to the rectal stump like small bowel or ureter. The main difficulty of this technique can be performing the transanal dissection in patients with hard adhesions to the rectal stump after perforation or peritonitis. Furthermore, a very short rectal stump makes positioning the transanal single-port access difficult and without adequate workspace impossible.

7. Authors' recommendation

The authors believe that the minimally invasive technique is an attractive approach for rever-sal of Hartmann's procedure. So far, reports are promising. The technique may reduce the substantial morbidity known from open reversal. The SIR technique may be considered to be obsolete, especially in the era of laparoscopy. Most patients will be best suited by use of lapa-roscopic techniques. We would like to emphasize that laparoscopy is a means to an end and not a goal in itself. If minimally invasive techniques are deemed unsafe or unsuitable, conver-sion to open technique may be utilized at any time. We believe that. The recently developed technique of single port restoration of continuity seems especially promising, as contralateral access that can be cumbersome due to the adhesions from a previous laparotomy is avoided and a ventral hernia defect when present can be avoided. We believe Trephine assess in combination with the transanal approach as primary surgical approach is not always necessary. We recommend this technique to be used as a step-up approach or back-up when pelvic dissection is proving technically challenging

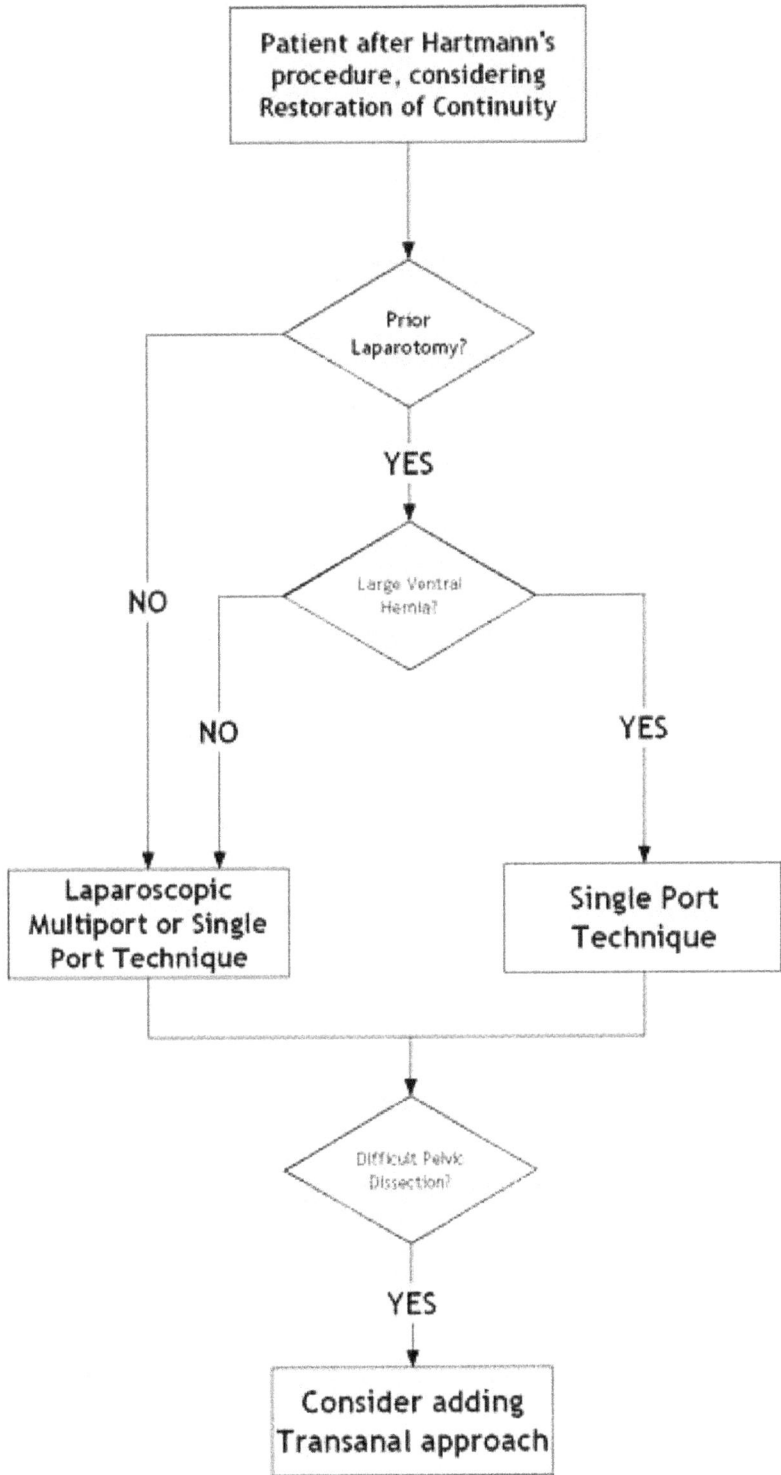

Figure 13. Algorithm to be used during the decision-making which technique is best suited for the restoration of bowel continuity after Hartmann's procedure.

or unsafe during initial trephine or multiport access. Authors recommendations are summarized in the algorithm in **Figure 13**.

8. Conclusion

The reversal of Hartmann's procedure carries a high operative morbidity and mortality rate. Therefore this is only performed in a selected group of patients. A considerable group of patients, with advanced age, or expected high operative risk, are left with a permanent end colostomy. This chapter gives an overview of the development less invasive techniques, that may reduce morbidity and therefore be offered to a larger group of patients.

Conventional laparoscopic reversal of Hartmann's procedure was the first technique with the primary goal of reducing morbidity and mortally. This technique reduced surgical access trauma resulting in a shorter post operative hospital stay and avoiding the negative consequences of relaparotomy. In the quest for even less invasive ways of restoring the bowel continuity the Trephine access technique was developed. This technique received criticism on the fact that the adhesiolysis was performed mainly in a blind fashion. This is probably the reason why this technique has not gained wide popularity and acceptance. This technique however gave birth to the development of the single-port access technique. This minimally invasive laparoscopic technique has our preference. We recommend using this technique for the major reduction in access trauma. Avoiding crossing the midline reduces the need for adhesiolysis, with its potential hazards like iatrogenic bowel injury. When proven safe in larger series, reversal of Hartmann's procedure may be offered to a larger proportion of patients then is presently routine.

Author details

Stefan H.E.M. Clermonts[1], Laurents P.S. Stassen[2] and David D.E. Zimmerman[1,*]

*Address all correspondence to: d.zimmerman@etz.nl

1 Department of Surgery, Elisabeth-TweeSteden Hospital, Tilburg, The Netherlands

2 Department of Surgery, Maastricht University Medical Center, Maastricht, The Netherlands

References

[1] Van Gulik TM, Mallonga ET, Taat CW. Henri Hartmann, Lord of the Hotel-Dieu. Nether J Surg. 1986(3):45–7.

[2] JP. Portraits de Chirurgiens de l'Hotel-Dieu. Presse Med. 1959(60):2317–20.

[3] Ronel DN, Hardy MA. Henri Albert Hartmann: labor and discipline. Curr Surg. 2002;59(1):59–64.

[4] HH. Nouveau procede d'ablation des cancers de la partie terminale du colon pelvien. Strasbourg: Trentienne Congres de Chirurgie, 1921:411–3.

[5] HH. Note sur un procede nouveau d'extripation des cancers de la partie terminale du colon. Bulletin et Memoires de la Societe Chirurgique de Paris. 1923:1474–7.

[6] Abbas S. Resection and primary anastomosis in acute complicated diverticulitis, a systematic review of the literature. Int J Colorectal Dis. 2007;22(4):351–7.

[7] Pearce NW, Scott SD, Karran SJ. Timing and method of reversal of Hartmann's procedure. Br J Surg. 1992;79(8):839–41.

[8] Wigmore SJ, Duthie GS, Young IE, Spalding EM, Rainey JB. Restoration of intestinal continuity following Hartmann's procedure: the Lothian experience 1987–1992. Br J Surg. 1995;82(1):27–30.

[9] Albarran SA, Simoens C, Van De Winkel N, da Costa PM, Thill V. Restoration of digestive continuity after Hartmann's procedure: ASA score is a predictive factor for risk of postoperative complications. Acta Chir Belg. 2009;109(6):714–9.

[10] Banerjee S, Leather AJ, Rennie JA, Samano N, Gonzalez JG, Papagrigoriadis S. Feasibility and morbidity of reversal of Hartmann's. Colorectal Dis: Off J Assoc Coloproctol G B Irel. 2005;7(5):454–9.

[11] Maggard MA, Zingmond D, O'Connell JB, Ko CY. What proportion of patients with an ostomy (for diverticulitis) get reversed? Am Surg. 2004;70(10):928–31.

[12] Nugent KP, Daniels P, Stewart B, Patankar R, Johnson CD. Quality of life in stoma patients. Dis Colon Rectum. 1999;42(12):1569–74.

[13] Mols F, Lemmens V, Bosscha K, van den Broek W, Thong MS. Living with the physical and mental consequences of an ostomy: a study among 1-10-year rectal cancer survivors from the population-based PROFILES registry. Psychooncology. 2014. Sep;23(9):998–1004.

[14] Roque-Castellano C, Marchena-Gomez J, Hemmersbach-Miller M, Acosta-Merida A, Rodriguez-Mendez A, Farina-Castro R, et al. Analysis of the factors related to the decision of restoring intestinal continuity after Hartmann's procedure. Int J Colorectal Dis. 2007;22(9):1091–6.

[15] Machairas A, Liakakos T, Patapis P, Petropoulos C, Tsapralis D, Misiakos EP. Prosthetic repair of incisional hernia combined with elective bowel operation. Surgeon: J R Coll Surg Edinb Irel. 2008;6(5):274–7.

[16] Seo SI, Lee JL, Park SH, Ha HK, Kim JC. Assessment by using a water-soluble contrast enema study of radiologic leakage in lower rectal cancer patients with sphincter-saving surgery. Ann Coloproctol. 2015;31(4):131–7.

[17] Kalady MF, Mantyh CR, Petrofski J, Ludwig KA. Routine contrast imaging of low pelvic anastomosis prior to closure of defunctioning ileostomy: is it necessary? J Gastrointest Surg. 2008;12(7):1227–31.

[18] Hong SY, Kim do Y, Oh SY, Suh KW. Routine barium enema prior to closure of defunctioning ileostomy is not necessary. J Korean Surg Soc. 2012;83(2):88–91.

[19] Keck JO, Collopy BT, Ryan PJ, Fink R, Mackay JR, Woods RJ. Reversal of Hartmann's procedure: effect of timing and technique on ease and safety. Dis Colon Rectum. 1994;37(3):243–8.

[20] Roe AM, Prabhu S, Ali A, Brown C, Brodribb AJ. Reversal of Hartmann's procedure: timing and operative technique. Br J Surg. 1991;78(10):1167–70.

[21] Kwon S, Morris A, Billingham R, Frankhouse J, Horvath K, Johnson M, et al. Routine leak testing in colorectal surgery in the Surgical Care and Outcomes Assessment Program. Arch Surg. 2012;147(4):345–51.

[22] Aydin HN, Remzi FH, Tekkis PP, Fazio VW. Hartmann's reversal is associated with high postoperative adverse events. Dis Colon Rectum. 2005;48(11):2117–26.

[23] Carcoforo P, Navarra G, Di Marco L, Occhionorelli S, Rocca T, Pollinzi V. Reversal of Hartmann's procedure. Our experience. Ann Ital Chir. 1997;68(4):523–7; discussion 7–8.

[24] Rosen MJ, Cobb WS, Kercher KW, Sing RF, Heniford BT. Laparoscopic restoration of intestinal continuity after Hartmann's procedure. Am J Surg. 2005;189(6):670–4.

[25] Faure JP, Doucet C, Essique D, Badra Y, Carretier M, Richer JP, et al. Comparison of conventional and laparoscopic Hartmann's procedure reversal. Surg Laparosc Endosc Percutan Tech. 2007;17(6):495–9.

[26] Haughn C, Ju B, Uchal M, Arnaud JP, Reed JF, Bergamaschi R. Complication rates after Hartmann's reversal: open vs. laparoscopic approach. Dis Colon Rectum. 2008;51(8):1232–6.

[27] Vermeulen J, Coene PP, Van Hout NM, van der Harst E, Gosselink MP, Mannaerts GH, et al. Restoration of bowel continuity after surgery for acute perforated diverticulitis: should Hartmann's procedure be considered a one-stage procedure? Colorectal Dis. 2009;11(6):619–24.

[28] Mazeh H, Greenstein AJ, Swedish K, Nguyen SQ, Lipskar A, Weber KJ, et al. Laparoscopic and open reversal of Hartmann's procedure—a comparative retrospective analysis. Surg Endosc. 2009;23(3):496–502.

[29] Di Carlo I, Toro A, Pannofino O, Patane E, Pulvirenti E. Laparoscopic versus open restoration of intestinal continuity after Hartmann procedure. Hepatogastroenterology. 2010;57(98):232–5.

[30] De'angelis N, Brunetti F, Memeo R, Batista da Costa J, Schneck AS, Carra MC, et al. Comparison between open and laparoscopic reversal of Hartmann's procedure for diverticulitis. World J Gastrointest Surg. 2013;5(8):245–51.

[31] Yang PF, Morgan MJ. Laparoscopic versus open reversal of Hartmann's procedure: a retrospective review. ANZ J Surg. 2014;84(12):965–9.

[32] Vermeulen J VW, Mannaerts GH, . Reversal of Hartmann's procedure through the stomal side: a new even more minimal invasive technique. Surg Endosc 2008;22(10):2319–22.

[33] van de Wall BJ, Draaisma WA, Schouten ES, Broeders IA, Consten EC. Conventional and laparoscopic reversal of the Hartmann procedure: a review of literature. J Gastrointest Surg. 2010;14(4):743–52.

[34] Vermeulen J., LJWA, Mannaerts GHH. Reversal of Hartmann's procedure after perforated diverticulitis through the stomal side without additional incisions: the SIR procedure. Dig Surg. 2010;27:391–6.

[35] Aydin C, Olmez A, Isik S, Sumer F, Kayaalp C. Reversal of the Hartmann procedure through only a stomal orifice. Am Surg. 2011;77(6):694–6.

[36] Parkin E, Khurshid M, Ravi S, Linn T. Surgical access through the stoma for laparoscopic reversal of Hartmann procedures. Surg Laparosc Endosc Percutan Tech. 2013;23(1):41–4.

[37] Clermonts SH, de Ruijter WM, van Loon YT, Wasowicz DK, Heisterkamp J, Maring JK, et al. Reversal of Hartmann's procedure utilizing single-port laparoscopy: an attractive alternative to laparotomy. Surg Endosc. 2016;30(5):1894–901.

[38] Borowski DW, Kanakala V, Agarwal AK, Tabaqchali MA, Garg DK, Gill TS. Single-port access laparoscopic reversal of Hartmann operation. Dis Colon Rectum. 2011;54(8):1053–6.

[39] Carus T, Emmert A. Single-port laparoscopic reversal of Hartmann's procedure: technique and results. Minim Invasive Surg 2011;2011:356784.

[40] Choi BJ, Jeong WJ, Kim YK, Kim SJ, Lee SC. Single-port laparoscopic reversal of Hartmann's procedure via the colostomy site. Int J Surg 2015;14:33–7.

[41] Joshi HM, Gosselink MP, Adusumilli S, Cunningham C, Lindsey I, Jones OM. Incisionless reversal of Hartmann's procedure. Tech Coloproctol. 2014;18(9):843–6.

[42] Smith BM, Bettinger DA. Single-incision laparoscopic reversal of Hartmann procedure via the colostomy site only: first report. Surg Innov. 2011;18(4):NP5–7.

[43] Bravo R, Fernandez-Hevia M, Jimenez-Toscano M, Flores LF, de Lacy B, Quaresima S, et al. Transanal Hartmann reversal: a new technique. Surg Endosc. 2016;30(6):2628–31.

4

Laparoscopic Appendectomy

Paolo Ialongo, Giuseppe Carbotta and
Antonio Prestera

Abstract

Appendectomy represents a fundamental step in the training course of a surgeon in so much that for several decades it has been the first surgical operation assigned to a training surgeon. Yet, laparoscopic appendectomy has not spread with the same characteristics as the operation of cholecystectomy for which laparoscopy has rapidly become the gold standard. We can moreover note that nowadays, in spite of a certain initial distrust, the laparoscopic methodology is fully employed in the treatment of acute appendicitis, even though the use of such technique is controversial in cases of acute complicated appendicitis.

Keywords: appendicitis, surgery, laparoscopy

1. Introduction

Appendectomy represents a fundamental step in the training course of a surgeon in so much that for several decades it has been the first surgical operation assigned to a training surgeon.

Yet, laparoscopic appendectomy has not spread with the same characteristics as the operation of cholecystectomy for which laparoscopy has rapidly become the gold standard.

In fact, before attempting their laparoscopic appendectomies, many surgeons have, first, standardised their technique of cholecystectomy. There are many reasons that justify a slower spreading of this methodology:

- Open appendectomy has been considered for decades as a rapid technical method requiring a small surgical incision.

- The operation is, moreover, generally made on an organ suffering from an inflammatory process which often causes a pathological alteration of the surrounding organs with formation of oedema, congestion and adhesions, thus making a laparoscopic appendectomy more difficult.

The open appendectomy introduced by an American surgeon Charles McBurney in 1894 is still today considered the gold standard in the surgical treatment of acute appendicitis because it is a safe surgical procedure, with a low morbidity rate, a short hospitalisation and a low discomfort for the patients. Expected intraoperative difficulties in laparoscopic appendectomy could be the management of peritonitis grade and of ectopic appendix.

The first video-assisted appendectomy seems to have been performed in 1977 by the Dutchman Hans J. De Kok, whose priority is actually unknown owing to the scanty circulation of the medical review which was published.

It was Kurt Semm, a German gynaecologist, who publicised the technique of a laparoscopic appendectomy in his two successive works (June 1982 and January 1983). Semm did not however consider the laparoscopic procedure fit for the case of acute appendicitis, as he confirmed in one of his articles published on the review "Endoscopy" in 1983. But he did not quote any personal case history or experience, thus exposing himself to much criticism.

Actually, in 1987 his countryman Jorg H. Schreiber, from Dusseldorf, published his first dense report of 70 cases in 5 years (of which 67 are made with the laparoscopic technique; 7 with a clinical picture of acute, catarrhal or phlegmonous appendicitis), claiming that he had performed his first laparoscopic appendectomy in June 1982.

The number of publications has been in constant growth since then, and more and more numerous perspective comparative studies show the validity and the safety of the laparoscopic procedure offering such significant advantages as fewer infections of the wound, reduced administration of analgesics and a faster return to normal activity, whereas some authors report that costs are increased and operative time are supposed to be longer than the open procedure.

We can moreover note that nowadays, in spite of a certain initial distrust, the laparoscopic methodology is fully employed in the treatment of acute appendicitis, even though the use of such technique is controversial in cases of acute complicated appendicitis.

Notwithstanding, of the numerous studies that have been published on this subject, there is not yet scientific evidence of the superiority of the laparoscopic technique [1] over the open surgical operation even though the laparoscopic procedure proves to be safe also in complicated case with diffuse peritonitis; in which cases it also allows to perform an accurate lavage of the abdominal cavity.

Despite each patient needs to be evaluated for the best surgical procedure, there is no absolute contraindication to laparoscopic appendectomy in cases of complicated appendicitis, especially for experienced surgeons, because it has been demonstrated that the patients in those cases gain a better postoperative outcome.

Open appendectomy presents a higher incidence of complications (wound infections, which can cause longer hospitalisation) and later postoperative hernias.

Laparoscopic procedure can assure a complete exploration of abdominal cavity, without a bigger incision and in case of ectopic or complicated appendicitis. In those cases, if conversion is needed, it could be possible that a focused incision can be practised. Mini-invasive technique is also useful to treat other associated diseases (previously referred or diagnosed during the surgery).

Among all advantages, described in literature, we must remember the reduction of wound infection incidence, of adhesion-related disorders (very important in young women because of infertility that can be caused by adhesions post appendicitis or salpingitis) and of postoperative pain, a faster hospitalisation, a quick return to daily activity and good aesthetic results.

For all these reasons, laparoscopic appendectomy seems to be destined to become unanimously the gold standard for the treatment of acute complicated appendectomy, just as it happened to laparoscopic cholecystectomy.

2. Epidemiology

Acute appendicitis manifests itself at all ages, mostly during infancy and adolescence; it mainly interests the male sex and has an annual incidence of 0.2%. About 14% of the population is estimated to get acute appendicitis during their lifetime. An early diagnosis and its urgent surgical operation are fundamentals to prevent complications and morbidity.

3. Indications

The advantages of a mini-invasive approach evidence themselves above all among women in childbearing age in whom the differential diagnosis is greatly improved. In this way the diagnosis of such pelvic pathologies which may fake an appendicitis as endometriosis, salpingitis and complications of ovarian cysts like torsions or ruptures of haemorrhagic corpus luteum is made possible, thus reducing the percentage of "innocent" appendicitis, as important meta-analyses clearly show [2]. The diagnostic advantage among children and members of the male sex seems to be less, since in this subgroup of patients the diagnosis of appendicitis and the probable differential diagnosis are simpler; anyway, a considerable percentage of cases (5.5%) is recorded where the diagnosis is modified and corrected by resorting to the laparoscopic technique [2]. In obese patients the postoperative complications of a laparoscopic appendectomy are fewer than those with an open technique. The laparoscopic methodology is applicable also to elderly patients, subject to preoperative diagnosis and in the absence of side effects in general. In literature there seems to be some advantage in favour of laparoscopic appendectomy; a more accurate preoperative diagnostic workup is anyway advised in consideration also of the greater incidence of neoplasias among elderly people [1, 3, 4]. There is no unanimous agreement about laparoscopic appendectomy on pregnant women. The most recent studies on this topic, though they consider the second 3 months as the safest period, do not warn against it during the other periods. Anyway, considering the relative benefits, as well as the potential risks (increase of mortality of foetuses), basing on the data recorded in literature, it is not advisable to prefer laparoscopic appendectomy during all the 3 months of pregnancy [1, 5, 6]. If at the laparoscopic exploration the appendix is shown to be macroscopically undamaged and another pathology is found out as the cause of the symptomatology, there is sufficient evidence that the appendix should not be removed. The difference is the case in which the appendix is normal, but no other pathology is found out; concerning this, it is worthwhile remembering the objective at difficulty, in some cases, of performing a macroscopic diagnosis of appendicitis. In fact an appendix under an initial inflammatory process may have a normal aspect but may result pathologically in the final histological examination. In such cases the surgeon shall decide case by case, on the basis of the preoperative clinical picture. The greater number of authors is in favour of exeresis, also in consideration of the improvement of the clinic symptomatology of such cases. In case of a complicated appendicitis, resorting to the laparoscopic approach is a questionable matter. According to the data recorded in literature, laparoscopy is feasible with the same amount of morbidity as with open technique, in spite of the increase of the incidence of intra-abdominal abscesses which are, on the other hand, counterbalanced by a minor incidence of infections of the wound. The greater incidence of postoperative abscesses may depend either on the relative inexperience of the surgeon or on defects in the surgical technique. The postoperative outcome in terms of total morbidity, hospitalisation and return to work seems, however, to be significantly better among patients with complicated appendicitis treated with the laparoscopic technique. As a matter of principle, the presence of peritonitis, of an abscess, of a gangrenous appendicitis or of perforation does not represent an indication to conversion to laparotomy. Each case must be judged separately, on the basis of the surgical and laparoscopic experience of the surgeon. Conversion to laparotomy is, however, advisable; any time the surgeon does not consider it safe to carry on the surgical operation by laparoscopy, and in such cases, it appears reasonable to make use of an access sufficiently large as to allow to explore and wash the abdominal cavity in an adequate way [7–10].

4. Surgical technique

4.1. Position of the patient

The patient is laid on his back on the surgical bed, with joined and blocked limbs. The right arm is extended laterally (abduction at 90°) so as to allow the anaesthetist's easy vascular access as well as the checking of the vital parameters; the left arm, completely abducted, is fixed to the body. During the surgical operation, some changes of position may be necessary (Trendelenburg, anti-Trendelenburg, left or right lateral inclination) which imply a good anchorage of the patient to the operative table, as accurately as the gravity of the clinical picture requires. In case of serious peritonitis, in fact, washing of the peritoneal cavity is made easier by varying the position of the patient.

4.2. Positioning of the team

The surgical team is made up of the surgeon, the assistant and the instrumentalist operator. This one must stand on the left side of the patient with the surgeon on his right, while the assistant, initially on the right of the patient, shall also move to the left between the surgeon and the instrument operator, after the insertion of the trocars. The service table is laid on the feet of the patient, on the left of the instrumentalist operator.

4.3. Positioning of the trocars

Umbilical, above pubis and in the left iliac fossa are considered the best ports so as to permit an optimal triangulation (**Figure 1**).

The Italian surgical school unanimously favours the technique of three trocars centred in the left hemi-abdomen as described in the early 1990s. The strong points of this position are the easiness of vision and of triangulation, but there is no evidence in literature of an improvement

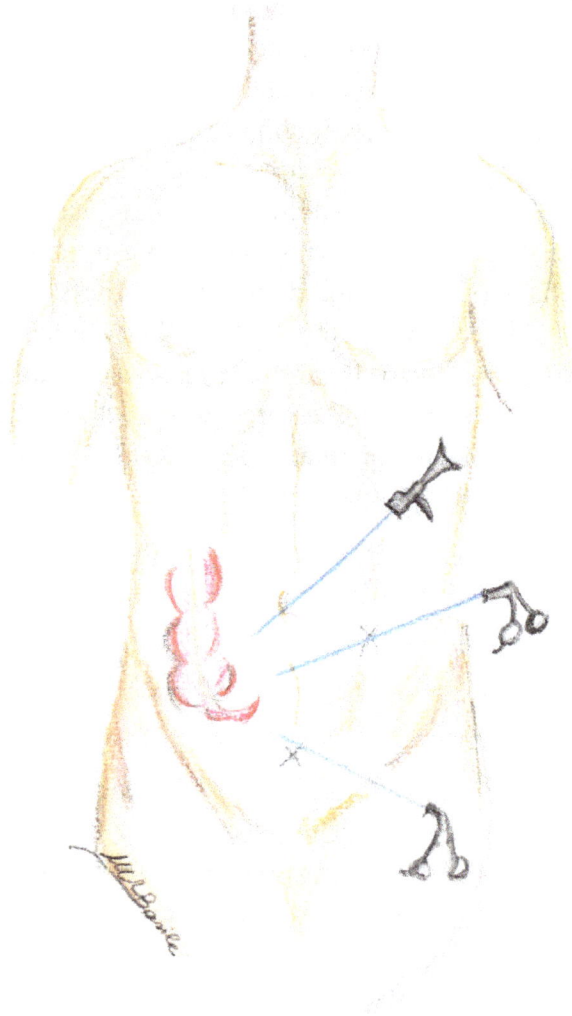

Figure 1. Positioning of the trocars.

of the outcome in comparison with other laparoscopic ports. The insertion of the second trocar in the region above pubis can sometimes present some difficulties; the parietal peritoneum may in fact easily come off the muscle planes, so the needle of the trocar does not pierce it completely but carries it into the abdominal cavity. It is therefore advisable while controlling the manoeuvre through the optical device on the first trocar to carry out the positioning of the trocar in the left iliac fossa as second positioning and not as third positioning; through the iliac trocar, a tenaculum can be introduced so as to press the parietal peritoneum outwards, thus facilitating its penetration. Some surgeons prefer to place the bladder catheter before introducing the trocar above the pubis region to empty the bladder to avoid iatrogenic damages. The use of the two trocars has been studied retrospectively, without evidencing significant advantages. The "single-port" technique has been described in some studies that have shown reduction of the surgical trauma, of the pain and of the postoperative stay in bed, as well as better aesthetic results, but there are still few evidences that it can be an adequate alternative to the standard laparoscopic technique, just as it is the case both with the micro-laparoscopic technique and with the NOTE technique (natural translumenal endoscopic surgery) which makes use of the transvaginal port.

4.4. Exploration of the abdominal cavity

As usual, in all surgical operations either laparoscopic or open, at the start, a careful exploration of the abdominal cavity is necessary with the aim of confirming the diagnosis and/or evidencing other problems. Then, with two atraumatic tenacula (Johanne type), the appendix is searched for by locating the caecum and then the terminal iliac loop. Sometimes, the appendix may take an unusual position (back to the caecum, go down into the Douglas cavity or be adherent to the abdominal wall). In such cases its finding may result difficult. Once the appendix is located, it must be isolated from possible inflammatory-type adhesions.

4.5. Coagulation and section of the meso-appendix

We take note of the great variety of possible usable devices, and we consider bipolar coagulation of the preferable method for the section of the meso-appendix because it is safer and cost-effective (**Figure 2**), even though more rapid, efficient and even more costly methods (e.g. ultrasounds) have been the subject of studies in literature. The appendix is tightened by means of Johanne-type tenacula, and with the chosen device, the meso-appendix is coagulated, starting from the free side towards the appendicular base. Much attention must be paid close to the appendicular artery which must be tied up and sectioned (either directly by means of electricity or by using two clips).

4.6. Tying up the appendicular base

The appendicular stump is closed up by positioning the loop (**Figure 3**), following the methodology already described by Semm in 1983; the mechanical endoscopic stitcher, the stapler, is an alternative approach much employed recently. When using loops, two of them are placed at the base, a few millimetres one from the other. When the stapler is employed, it must comprise the base of the appendix with a piece of caecum as large as a stamp to ensure safe

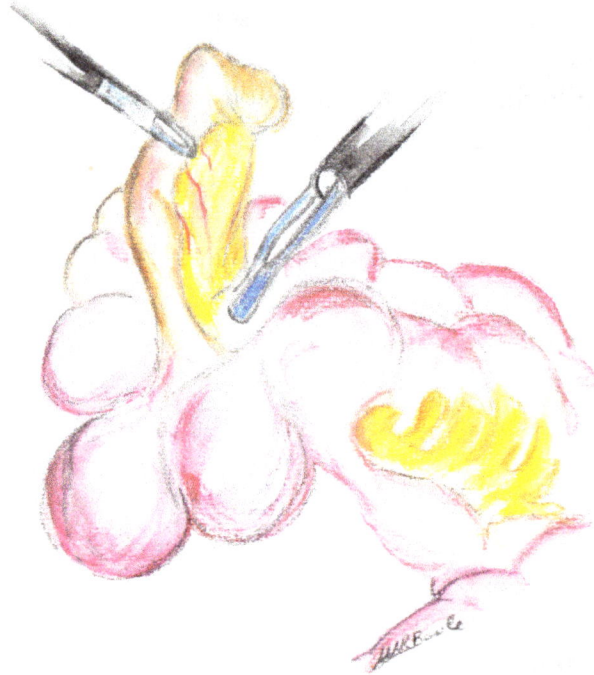

Figure 2. Coagulation and section of the meso-appendix.

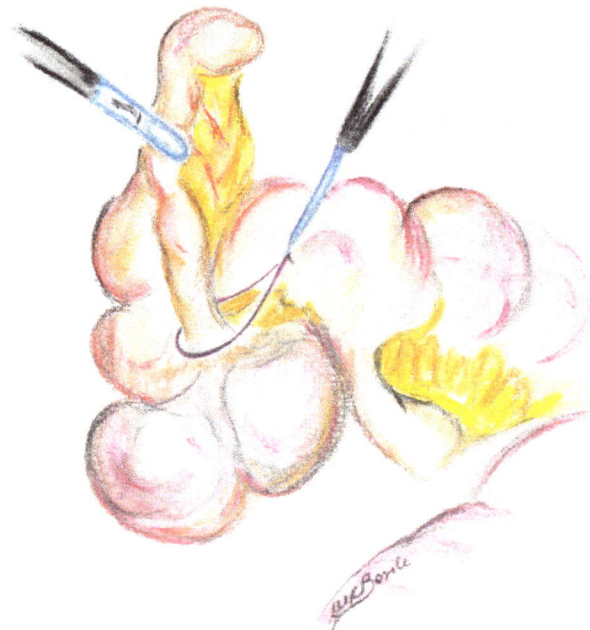

Figure 3. Tying up of the appendicular base.

closure. Numerous comparative studies have been published about these two approaches. Those in favour of the use of a stapler underline such advantages of this technique as the possibility of using it even in complicated appendicitis, reduction of the operating time and of the formation of endo-abdominal abscesses and a fast post-operation canalization of faeces not to mention the easy use on the part of training surgeons. The authors in favour of the use of loops point out an unmeaningful difference between the two techniques, except for the operating time. The looping technique is considered also a good exercise of manual skill for young surgeons and an economic aid, differently from the stapler which, for the same reason, is not economic for a systematic use [1, 11]. The disadvantages of using the loop are, instead, represented by the large learning curve as well as by its not-yet-clear role in complicated appendicitis [1]. In sectioning the viscera, an adequate length of the residual stump is recommended, which inside must be free of coprolites. Appendicitis of the stump is a rare entity but much attention must be paid to the remaining part of the appendix to minimise such a complication [12]. To further reduce costs, some authors advise to make use of reabsorbing clips (hem-o-lok) to suture the appendix but only in the catarrhal forms.

4.7. Removal of the appendix

It is recommended in all cases to protect the abdominal wall accurately during the extraction of the viscera, either by means of endo-bags, by extraction within the trocar or by other aids which may avoid contamination. Infections of wound are remarkably reduced with the laparoscopic appendectomy thanks to the routine use of protection of the operating piece during the extraction. In those cases in which protection is not employed (e.g., in the so-called laparo-assisted one trocar technique), the incidence of postoperative infections rises up to levels which can be compared to those of the open technique [13]. In case of widespread peritonitis, abscess or perforated appendix, a complete peritoneal washing is recommended. The fact of finding postoperative intra-abdominal abscesses in noncomplicated appendix laparoscopically treated has raised the doubt that limited and aimed washing may reduce the incidence, even if only one retrospective study supports this hypothesis [14, 15]. Therefore, in cases of localised phlogosis, aspiration of the effusions by means of localised washing is considered a protective measure against spreading the septic content towards the recesses unharmed by phlogosis. The routine use of drainage is not advisable; it can, however, be useful for therapeutic purposes either in the presence of abscess cavity and of widespread peritonitis [16] or for preventive treatment in particular situations of risk (steroidal therapy, chronic pathologies) and in special patients. In the other cases, the use of drainage is not necessary and can even be harmful.

Author details

Paolo Ialongo[1]*, Giuseppe Carbotta[1] and Antonio Prestera[1,2]

*Address all correspondence to: ialongopaolo@gmail.com

1 General Surgery Unit, Department of Emergency and Organ Transplantation, School of Medicine, "Aldo Moro", University of Bari, Bari, Italy

2 Surgery Unit, Hospital of Gallipoli, Lecce, Italy

References

[1] Gorter RR, Heij HA, Eker HH, Kazemier G. Laparoscopic appendectomy: State of the art. Tailored approach to the application of laparoscopic appendectomy? Best Practice & Research. Clinical Gastroenterology. February 2014;28(1):211-224

[2] Tzvoras G, Liakou P, Baloyiannis I, et al. Laparoscopic appendectomy: Differences between male and female patients with suspected acute appendicitis. World Journal of Surgery. 2007;31:409-413

[3] Baek HN, Jung YH, Hwang YH. Laparoscopic versus open appendectomy for appendicitis in elderly patient. Journal of the Korean Society of Coloproctology. 2011;27(5):241-245

[4] Kirshtein B, Perry ZH, Mizrahi S, Lantsberg L. Value of laparoscopic appendectomy in the elderly patient. World Journal of Surgery. 2009;33:918-922

[5] Jackson H, Granger S, Price R, et al. Diagnosis and laparoscopic treatment of surgical diseases during pregnancy: An evidence -based review. Surgical Endoscopy. 2008; 22:1917-1927

[6] Walsh CA, Tang T, Walsh SR. Laparoscopic versus open appendectomy in pregnancy: A systematic review. International Journal of Surgery. 2008;6:339-344

[7] Ferranti et al. Laparoscopic versus open appendectomy for the treatment of complicated appendicitis. Il Giornale di Chirurgia. 2012;33(8/9):263-267

[8] Lim SG, Jung Ahn E, Kim SY, Il YC, Park J-M, Choi S hY PKW. A clinical comparison of laparoscopic versus open appendectomy for complicated appendicitis. Journal of the Korean Society of Coloproctology. 2011;27(6):293-297

[9] Yau KK, Siu WT, Tang CN, et al. Laparoscopic versus open appendectomy for complicated appendicitis. Journal of the American College of Surgeons. 2007;205:60-65

[10] Cueto J, D'Allemagne B, Vazquez-Frias JA, et al. Morbidity of laparoscopic surgery for complicated appendicitis: An international study. Surgical Endoscopy. 2006;20:717-720

[11] Sajid MS, Rimple J, Cheek E, Baig MK. Uso de endo-GIA versus endo-loop for securing the appendicular stump in laparoscopic appendectomy: A systematic review. Surgical Laparoscopy, Endoscopy & Percutaneous Techniques. 2009;19:11-15

[12] Truty MJ, Stulak JM, Utter PA, et al. Appendicitis after appendectomy. Archives of Surgery. 2008;143:413-415

[13] Romy S, Eisering MC, Bettschart V, et al. Laparoscope use and surgical site infections in digestive surgery. Annals of Surgery. 2008;247:627-632

[14] Gupta R, Sample C, Barnehriz F, Birch DW. Infectious complications following laparoscopic appendectomy. Canadian Journal of Surgery. 2006;49:397-400

[15] Hussain A, Mhmood H, Nicholls J, El-Hasani S. Prevention of intra-abdominal abscess following laparoscopic appendectomy for perforated appendicitis: A prospective study. International Journal of Surgery. 2008;**6**:374-377

[16] Petrowsky H, Demartines N, Rousson V, Clavien PA. Evidence -based value of prophylactic drainage in gastrointestinal surgery. A systematic review and meta-analyses. Annals of Surgery. 2004;**240**:1074-1085

5

Laparoscopic Pancreas Surgery: Image Guidance Solutions

Juan A. Sánchez-Margallo, Thomas Langø,
Erlend F. Hofstad, Ronald Mårvik and
Francisco M. Sánchez-Margallo

Abstract

Pancreatic ductal adenocarcinoma (PDA) is the fourth leading cause of cancer-related deaths. Surgery is the only viable treatment, but irradical resection rates are still high. Laparoscopic pancreatic surgery has some technical limitations for surgeons and tumor identification may be challenging. Image-guided techniques provide intraoperative margin assessment and visualization methods, which may be advantageous in guiding the surgeon to achieve curative resections and therefore improve the surgical outcomes. In this chapter, current available laparoscopic surgical approaches and image-guided techniques for pancreatic surgery are reviewed. Surgical outcomes of pancreaticoduodenectomy and distal pancreatectomy performed by laparoscopy, laparoendoscopic single-site surgery (LESS), and robotic surgery are included and analyzed. Besides, image-guided techniques such as intraoperative near-infrared fluorescence imaging and surgical navigation are presented as emerging techniques. Results show that minimally invasive procedures reported a reduction of blood loss, reduced length of hospital stay, and positive resection margins, as well as an improvement in spleen-preserving rates, when compared to open surgery. Studies reported that fluorescence-guided pancreatic surgery might be beneficial in cases where the pancreatic anatomy is difficult to identify. The first approach of a surgical navigation system for guidance during pancreatic resection procedures is presented, combining preoperative images (CT and MRI) with intraoperative laparoscopic ultrasound imaging.

Keywords: pancreatic cancer, laparoendoscopic single-site surgery, robotic surgery, image-guided surgery, surgical navigation, near-infrared fluorescence

1. Introduction

Cancer is the second leading cause of death worldwide after heart disease, with 14.9 million cases and 8.2 million deaths in 2013 [1, 2] and the first leading cause of death among adults aged 40–79 years [3, 4]. Worldwide, pancreatic ductal adenocarcinoma (PDA) is the fourth leading cause of cancer-related deaths [2, 3]. The incidence of all types of pancreatic cancer ranges from 1 to 10 cases per 100,000 people and is generally higher in developed countries and among men [1, 2]. This has remained stable for the past 30 years relative to the incidence of other common solid tumors [5]. Each year about 233,000 new cases of pancreatic cancer are diagnosed worldwide [2, 3]. In the United States, the American Cancer Association expected about 48,960 (24,840 men and 24,120 women) cases of incidence in pancreatic cancer in 2015, with a mortality rate of 83% [6]. In Europe, the estimated number of new cases of pancreatic cancer in 2012 was 79,331 and the estimated number of cases of deaths was 78,669 [7, 8], which is almost the double than in the United States. The 5-year survival rate in the world for pancreatic cancer is still very low, with only 6%. In addition, the overall 2-year survival rate is less than 10%, which has hardly improved over the past two decades [3–5]. In fact, in contrast to the stable or declining trends for most cancer types in the United States, a trend analysis for 2001–2010 indicated that death rates are rising for pancreatic cancer [3, 4].

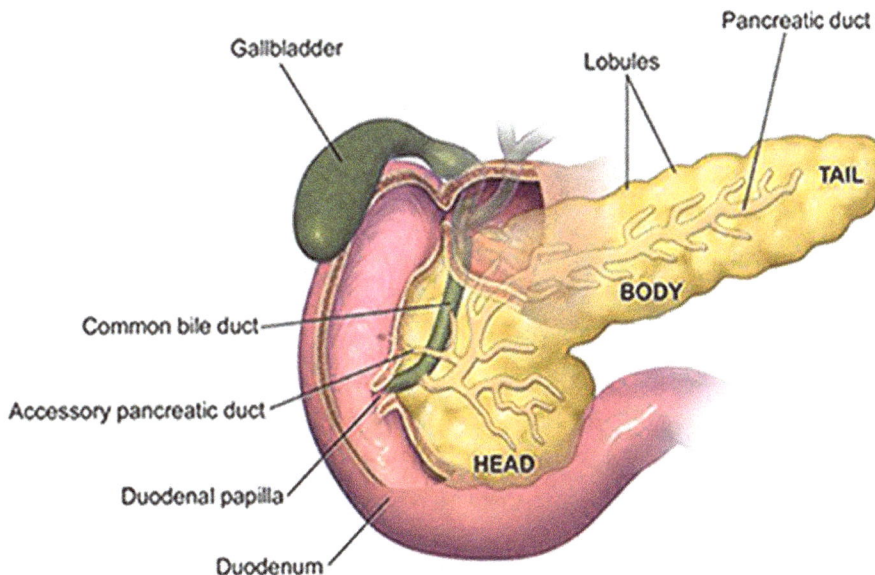

Figure 1. Anatomy of the pancreas. *Source:* "Blausen Gallery 2014". Wikiversity Journal of Medicine.

Pancreatic tumors are mainly classified as exocrine and endocrine tumors, also known as pancreatic neuroendocrine tumors (NETs). Exocrine tumors are approximately 99% of all primary pancreatic tumors [9] and are divided into ductal adenocarcinomas (80–90% of exocrine tumors), cystic neoplasms, and solid pseudopapillary neoplasms [5, 6, 10]. Ductal adenocarcinomas usually begin in the ducts of the pancreas and are located in the head of the pancreas (60–70%) (**Figure 1**) [10]. Approximately 5–10% of PDA cases are believed to be due to hereditary conditions, such as hereditary pancreatitis, Gardner syndrome, familial colon cancer, and others [11].

Pancreatic cases are usually diagnosed at an advanced stage but with few treatment options available. This is attributed primarily to a lack of reliable methods for early diagnosis and rapid metastasis of pancreatic cancer [12]. At the time of diagnosis, less than 20% of patients with pancreatic cancer present with localized, potentially curable tumors [13, 14]. Approximately, 30% of patients receive a diagnosis of advanced loco-regional disease. In addition, 30% of patients have local recurrence of tumors after treatment for an early disease [14].

Although there are several available treatments for pancreatic cancer such as ablative techniques, radiation therapies, and chemotherapy, surgery is the only viable treatment. However, only 10–20% of pancreatic tumors are candidates to be surgically resected at diagnosis [10, 15]. The required surgical intervention for pancreatic cancer treatment depends on the location of tumors. Cancers arising in the head of the pancreas require a pancreaticoduodenectomy (Whipple operation), while those in the tail require a distal pancreatectomy with or without splenectomy [16]. Lesions located in the neck and body may require a distal pancreatectomy, pancreaticoduodenectomy or, rarely, a total pancreatectomy. After surgery, patients with no positive resection margins (R0) have the most favorable prognosis [17]. The median survival length reported for resected (R0) pancreatic cancer ranges from 17–27 months and, after a R1 resection, the average survival length is 10.3 months [18]. However, irradical resection of pancreatic cancers still occurs in 35–42% of patients [16, 19]. This survival time is longer in patients with malignant disease localized to the pancreas and less than 3 cm in diameter than in patients with tumors of greater size or with retroperitoneal invasion (6–15 months) [13]. Other factors, such as tumor size, lymph node status, tumor grade and blood vessel invasion, are also correlated with prognosis [20].

The introduction of minimally invasive surgical techniques in the treatment of pancreatic cancer has allowed almost any pancreatic tumor to be operated by laparoscopic or robotic approaches with similar outcomes to the standard approach [21, 22]. Even new approaches such as laparosendoscopic single-site surgery (LESS) are being applied recently in the field of pancreatic surgery [23, 24]. However, there are some limitations that have hindered the wide use of minimally invasive pancreatic surgery, mainly due to the challenges of these kinds of interventions. The retroperitoneal location of the pancreas makes it difficult to reach during surgery. In addition, this glandular organ presents a delicate structure close to major vascular structures. There are also some technical limitations related to minimally invasive surgery (MIS) such as the lack of visual and tactile information. Increasing the capability to visualize tumor margins or to identify small metastatic nodules may significantly improve the surgical procedure to prevent positive resection margins, and therefore, surgical outcomes [25]. Image-guided techniques can provide intraoperative margin assessment and visualization methods, which may be advantageous in guiding the surgeon to achieve curative resections. Some of these emerging modalities are intraoperative near-infrared fluorescence imaging and surgical navigation systems [26, 27]. However, despite the high rate of positive resections in pancreatic surgery, there is limited medical literature regarding the use of navigation systems as a support during pancreatic interventions. In this chapter, the current laparoscopic surgical techniques and image-guided methods for pancreatic surgery and their associate surgical outcomes will be reviewed.

2. Laparoscopic techniques for pancreatic surgery

Pancreatic cancer is a complex disease, whose optimal treatment depends heavily on careful accurate staging [28]. Surgical resection is still the only potentially curative therapy for pancreatic cancer. However, pancreatic resection is technically challenging and a complex surgical procedure. In this section, the current laparoscopic surgical techniques for pancreatic surgery and their associated surgical outcomes will be reviewed. In order to reach more representative information, only studies published after 2010 and with more than 50 patients included, were taken into account. No limitation in the number of patients was set for the studies using LESS.

2.1. Laparoscopic surgery

2.1.1. Laparoscopic pancreaticoduodenectomy

The first laparoscopic pancreaticoduodenectomy (LPD) was published by Gagner and Pomp in 1994 [29]. They concluded that, although technically feasible, this approach did not confer significant benefit over the conventional open approach in terms of postoperative outcomes or reduced postoperative recovery period. One of the largest barriers of this complex procedure is the reconstruction phase due to the three separate anastomoses to be performed (pancreaticojejunostomy, hepaticojejunostomy, and gastrojejunostomy).

	N	Conv. (%)	Time (min)	EBL (ml)	LHS (days)	Morb. (%)	Mort. (%)	PF (%)	LN (%)	R0 (%)
[30]	53	17	541	195	8	77.3	5.7	13.2	44.2	94.9
[31]	384				10		5.2		4.7	80
[32]	983						5. 1			
[33]	108		379.4	492.4	6					
[34]	65	4.6	368	240	7	40	1.5	16.9	23.1	89
[35]	105	4.7	487.3		15	25	0.9	5.7	12.4	100
[36]	96	3.1					0	28.1		
[37]	75	13.3	551		7	31		9.3		
[38]	137		480.4	592	14.1					
[39]	681				9	39.4	3.8			

N: number of patients; Conv.: conversions; EBL: estimated blood loss; LHS: length of hospital stay; Morb.: morbidity rate; Mort.: mortality rate; PF: pancreatic fistulas; LN: lymph nodes; R0: R0 resection rate.

Table 1. Reported outcomes in laparoscopic pancreaticoduodenectomy.

A summary of the outcomes reported for LPDs are presented in **Table 1**. The average operation time was 486.7 min (range 368–551 min), 8.5% (range 3–17%) conversions, 342.3 ml (range 195–

592 ml) blood loss, 8.9 days (range 6–15 days) hospital stay, 32% (range 25–40%) morbidity, 2.6% (range 0–5%) mortality, 14.7% (range 6–28%) pancreatic fistulas, 21.1% (range 6–28%) harvested lymph nodes, and 89.7% (range 80–100%) R0 resection. The highest rate of conversions reported was due to suspected portal vein involvement [30]. Regarding morbidity rates, the highest rate was caused mainly by surgical site infection, postoperative pancreatic fistula, and intraabdominal access [30]. Myocardial infarctions and positive margins were the main mortality causes [30, 31]. Comparing these results with the conventional open approach [16], LPD leads to an increase in operating time, rate of pancreatic fistulas, and R0 resections; a decrease in estimated blood loss and harvested lymph nodes; and similar results in length of hospital stay, morbidity, and mortality rates.

Most of the studies reported longer operation times using the laparoscopic approach compared to the open approach [30, 35, 37]. Although some studies reported comparable outcomes between open and LPD [30], in general, reduction of blood loss and hospital stay [33, 34] are shown for LPD. In some studies, LPD was associated with equivalent overall hospital cost compared with open pancreaticoduodenectomy [37, 39]. While operating time and supply costs were higher for LPD, it was balanced by reduced cost due to the shorter postoperative hospital stay. A steep learning curve is another aspect associated with LDP and some researchers stated that this procedure should be performed in centers by surgeons with substantial knowledge, experience, and skills [34, 36].

2.1.2. Laparoscopic distal pancreatectomy

Laparoscopic distal pancreatectomy (LDP) was first reported in 1996 by Gagner and Cuschieri [40, 41]. During this intervention, the tail of the pancreas or the tail and a portion of the body of the pancreas are removed. In some cases, the spleen is also removed. This operation is used more often to treat pancreatic NETs found in the tail and body of the pancreas. The determination of resectability is often based on the extent of involvement of the celiac axis [42].

A summary of the outcomes for LDPs are shown in **Table 2**. In brief, the average operation time was 215.2 min, 12% conversion rate, 241.7 ml estimated blood loss, 7.6 days length of hospital stay, 32.5% morbidity rate, 0.3% mortality rate, 21.2% pancreatic fistulas, 10.2% harvested lymph nodes, 89.5% R0 resection, and 46.3% spleen-preserving rate. Comparing these results with the outcomes from conventional open surgery [43, 44], there is a decrease in operation time, estimated blood loss, length of hospital stay, and mortality rate; similar morbidity rates; and an increased rate of pancreatic fistulas and spleen preservation.

Satisfactory oncological outcomes have been reported for LDP in patients with PDA and left-side pancreatic neoplasms [58, 61]. Although some studies reported similar outcomes as open distal pancreatectomy [21], most of the studies reported a clear reduction of blood loss [50, 53, 62, 63, 65] and hospital stay [45, 48, 50, 53, 31, 59, 61–65]. An increase in quality of life is reported when compared to the conventional approach [46]. Similar costs for the laparoscopic and open approaches are reported [63]. The increased OR cost associated with LDP is often offset by the shorter hospitalization and lower overall cost of postoperative care [57].

Regarding the spleen-preserving rate, results stated that it is worth to attempt laparoscopic spleen-preserving DP in patients with a presumed benign to borderline tumor of the body-tail of the pancreas [54]. The most positive results were reported for the splenic vessels preservation technique regarding the conservation of the spleen [51, 66].

	N	Conv. (%)	Time (min)	EBL (ml)	LHS (days)	Morb. (%)	Mort. (%)	PF (%)	LN (%)	R0 (%)	SP (%)
[21]	64	32.8	213	275	8	16		11	8	62	79.6
[45]	535	22.8			7		0		15	86	
[46]	100	23	239	464	7.7	66	0	53		73.3	
[47]	94							0	11		
[48]	71	9.1	250	150	5	28.2	0	11		97.2	15.5
[49]	67	14.9	203	100	6	21	1.5	19	6		
[50]	107	30	193	150	5	27	0	15		97	21
[51]* †	55	9	214.7	342.8	8.2	27.3	0	16			93.4
[51]* †	85	13	199.2	288.9	10.5	38.8	0	26	3		84.7
[52]	132	6.1	156.5	197.4	6	43.2	0.8	21	8	96.2	9.8
[53]	131	31.3	193	262	5	32	0	8	11	100	22.1
[54]	100	2	207		8.7	49	0	27		98	41
[55]	143	5.6	236	334				17			
[56]	902	6.4	316	243	18.9	23.6		66	11		32
[57]	70	7.1	145	113	5.8	49	0	36	5		
[58]	196	2.5	220	250	8	31.9	0	24	10	83.8	
[59]	144	39.5			6.8		0		17	87	
[60]	70	7.1	239		9	25.7	0	19	3	75.7	
[61]	359		195		8	12	0	28	20	91.6	49.6
[62]	82	7	188	70	4	32.9	0	13		97	12
[63]	100	4	214	171	6.1	34	3	17	15	100	25
[64]	73	15	352		5	40	0	22		97	
[65]	45	0	158.7	122.6	7.9	26.7		16			53.3
[66]†	70	0	220	352	10.4	32.9	0	17			100
[67]* †	246	0	193.4	378	8.2	32.5	0	20			54.8
[67]* †	203	0	204.4	328	7.7	25	0	4			

N: number of patients; Conv.: conversions; EBL: estimated blood loss; LHS: length of hospital stay; Morb.: morbidity rate; Mort.: mortality rate; PF: pancreatic fistulas; LN: lymph nodes; R0: R0 resection rate; SP: spleen preserving.
*Two groups.
†Spleen-preserving DP.

Table 2. Reported outcomes in laparoscopic distal pancreatectomy.

With growing surgical experience and refinement in the surgical technique, the indications for LDP have substantially broadened [52]. In this sense, the learning curve appeared to have been completed after 17 procedures [68], but strict selection criteria, high-volume hospital, and experienced team in open pancreatic surgery may play an important role in shortening this learning curve [69].

2.2. Laparoendoscopic single-site surgery

Recent interest in improving cosmetic outcomes has led to laparoendoscopic single-site surgery (LESS) being performed in a variety of procedures. In this sense, LESS is now consolidated as a real alternative to conventional laparoscopic surgery, with numerous studies sustaining its feasibility and therapeutic safety. However, single-site pancreatectomy has been explored and described only in recent years, and therefore, literature is limited to DP procedures and mostly to single case reports or small case series, as it is considered to be a challenging procedure. Only one study has been found for a PD through the single-site approach [70]. In this case, a surgical resection for a malignant melanoma metastatic to the pancreas was performed. The resection was carried out preserving the pylorus. No detailed information about the intervention and surgical outcomes were reported.

	N	Conv. (%)	Time (min)	EBL (ml)	LHS (days)	Morb. (%)	Mort. (%)	PF (%)	LN (%)	R0 (%)	SP (%)
[23]	20		176		2	4	20	20	0	100	90
[24]	14	7.1	166.4	157.1	7.6	0	7.1	0			50
[71]	1	0	330	100	7	1		100	0	100	0
[72]	1	0	170		5		0			100	0
[73]†	1	0	233	<100	3		0			100	100
[74]	12	20	279.8	185	12.2	3		41.6	25	100	33.3
[75]	8	0	145	225	6	2		50	25	100	62.5
[76]*	2	0	232.5	100	7, 5		0	100			
[77]	1	0			5	0			0	100	0

N: number of patients; Conv.: conversions; EBL: estimated blood loss; LHS: length of hospital stay; Morb.: morbidity rate; Mort.: mortality rate; PF: pancreatic fistulas; LN: lymph nodes; R0: R0 resection rate; SP: spleen preserving.
*Two groups.
†Spleen-preserving DP.

Table 3. Reported outcomes in single-site distal pancreatectomy.

The average operation time reported for LESS distal pancreatectomy (**Table 3**) was 218 min (range 145–330 min), 3% (range 0–20%) conversion rate, 144 ml (range 100–225 ml) estimated blood loss, 6 days (range 2–12 days) length of hospital stay, 15% (range 0–50%) morbidity, 0% mortality, 100% R0 resection, and 42% (range 0–100) spleen-preserving rate. Comparing the results with the conventional laparoscopic approach, there is a decreased rate of conversions, estimated blood loss, length of hospital stay, and morbidity; a similar mortality rate; increased average of pancreatic fistulas and R0 resections; and lower spleen-preserving rate.

Barbaros et al. [71] reported the first transumbilical laparoscopic single-site DP in a patient with metastatic lesions on the pancreas. The patient developed a pancreatic fistula. Haugvik et al. [75] compared the results of 8 single-incision DPs with 16 conventional LDPs. They reported no significant differences in operative time, intraoperative bleeding, resection status, and hospital stay between the two groups. Four surgical complications were reported for LESS and five for the conventional approach, including two patients for each group who developed a pancreatic fistula. There was no conversion to conventional laparoscopic or open surgery in any procedure. No differences between operative and postoperative results were also obtained by Yao et al. [24], who compared the surgical outcomes of 14 transumbilical laparoscopic single-site DPs with seven conventional multiport interventions. One conversion to open surgery and one case of leakage were reported for the LESS interventions. Machado et al. [23] reported 4 cases of pancreatic fistula in a study of 20 DPs. Some cases reported no surgical complications during the intervention [72, 76]. In a case study without using any commercial surgical port for LESS [77], the patient developed fever and leukocytosis after surgery. Bracale et al. [72] presented the first LESS DP for an adenocarcinoma. They reported no postoperative complications after 4 months follow-up.

Spleen preservation is an important issue in patients undergoing DP. However, only a few studies have reported spleen preservation through LESS. Chang et al. [73] reported a case of ransumbilical LESS spleen-preserving DP for a cystic tumor in the body of the pancreas. No surgical complications were reported. In another study, Han et al. [74] compared the results from 12 LESS DPs to 28 cases using a conventional laparoscopic approach. The mean surgery time and hospital stay in the LESS group were significantly longer. The spleen preservation was possible in 60.7% of the patients who underwent the conventional approach and 33.3% for the LESS. No significant differences in intraoperative blood loss, tumor size, conversion rate, and postoperative complications between the two groups were found.

In general, authors stated that single-site laparoscopic PD is a feasible and safe technique [23, 72, 74], which can be successfully performed in selected cases and qualified centers [71, 73]. However, they also stated that it is a very demanding procedure with a steep learning curve [74].

2.3. Robotic surgery

Robotic platforms, as the da Vinci® Surgical System (Intuitive Surgical, Sunnyvale, CA, USA), try to overcome many of the key shortcomings of traditional laparoscopy that include monocular vision, limited degrees of freedom, and the effects of pivot and fulcrum, which make complex tasks difficult to master. However, there are also some drawbacks regarding the use of these systems such as the lack of tactile feedback and their cost, including mainte-nance. Since its first reported application in 2003 [78], the application of robotic technology in pancreatic interventions has been increasing. The main benefit of robotic-assisted PD in comparison with LPD may be the ease of intracorporeal reconstruction after a long resection [78].

In the scientific literature, most of the studies regarding the robotic-assisted PD and DP are retrospective reviews and case reports (**Table 4** and **5**). The average operation time reported for robot-assisted PD (**Table 4**) was 489.1 min (range 410–568 min), 10% (range 0–22%) conversion rate, 324 ml (range 250–400 ml) estimated blood loss, 13.4 days (range 9–22 days) hospital stay, 48.6% (range 21–67%) morbidity rate, 3.8% (range 1–7%) mortality rate, 17.4% (range 7–30) pancreatic fistulas, 29% (range 11–70%) harvested lymph nodes, and 91% (range 87–95%) R0 resection. Comparing the results with conventional laparoscopic approach, operative time, length of hospital stay, and negative resections margins are similar; the rate of conversions, morbidity, mortality, and pancreatic fistulas are increased. Positive results have been obtained for robotic-assisted PD in patients with aberrant or anomalous hepatic arterial anatomy [22]. In a prospective analysis with 150 patients, Polanco et al. [79] concluded that larger body mass index, higher EBL, smaller tumor size and smaller duct diameter are the main predictors of postoperative PF in robot-assisted PD. It appears that the learning curve for robot-assisted PD is attained within 80 cases [80].

	N	Conv. (%)	Time (min)	EBL (ml)	LHS (days)	Morb. (%)	Mort. (%)	PF (%)	LN (%)	R0 (%)
[22]*	112	0	500	250	9.5	63.3	6.7	7	20	92.6
[79]	150	7.3	515	300				17		
[80]	200	6.5	483	250	9	67.5	3.3	17	11	92
[84]	60		410	400	20	35	1.7	13	23	94.7
[85]	50	22	421	394	22			30	70	90
[86]	50	16	568	350	10	56	2	20	36	89
[87]	132	8.3	527	>400	10	21	5.3	17	14	87.7

N: number of patients; Conv.: conversions; EBL: estimated blood loss; LHS: length of hospital stay; Morb.: morbidity rate; Mort.: mortality rate; PF: pancreatic fistulas; LN: lymph nodes; R0: R0 resection rate; SP: spleen preserving. *Two groups.

Table 4. Reported outcomes in robotic-assisted pancreaticoduodenectomy.

	N	Conv. (%)	Time (min)	EBL (ml)	LHS (days)	Morb. (%)	Mort. (%)	PF (%)	LN (%)	R0 (%)	SP (%)
[45]	535	23			7				3	86	
[82]	100	2	246	150		72	0	42	13	95.7	
[83]	55	0	278.2		12.6	61.8	0	53	58	100	61.8
[87]	83	2.4	256	>200	6	13	0	43	17	97	
[88]†	69	0	150	100	11.6	40.6	0	25	22	100	65.2

N: number of patients; Conv.: conversions; EBL: estimated blood loss; LHS: length of hospital stay; Morb.: morbidity rate; Mort.: mortality rate; PF: pancreatic fistulas; LN: lymph nodes; R0: R0 resection rate; SP: spleen preserving. †Spleen-preserving DP.

Table 5. Reported outcomes in robotic-assisted distal pancreatectomy.

Regarding robot-assisted DP, the average operation time was 232.6 min (range 150–278 min), 5.5% (range 0–23%) conversion rate, 125 ml (range 100–150 ml) estimated blood loss, 9.3 days (range 6–13 days) hospital stay, 46.9% (range 13–72%) morbidity rate, 0% mortality rate, 40.7% (range 24–53%) pancreatic fistula, 22.6% (range 3–58%) harvested lymph nodes, 95.7% (range 86–100%) R0 resection, and 63.5% (range 62–65%) spleen-preserving rate. Comparing these results with the conventional laparoscopic approach, there is a decreased conversion rate and EBL; and increased operation time, length of hospital stay, morbidity, rate of pancreatic fistulas, R0 resections, and spleen-preserving rate. Morbid obesity and technical difficulty seem to be the two most common reasons for conversion from robotic-assisted hepatobiliary and pancreatic surgery [81]. It appears that the learning curve for robot-assisted DP is approximately 10–40 cases [82, 83].

3. Image-guided techniques for pancreatic surgery

In order to cope with some of the limitations in MIS and guide the surgeon during the surgical procedure, image-guided techniques have been developed. The lack of tactile feedback and 3D sensation in video-assisted surgery accelerated the need for these techniques. In addition, for the human eye, several pathologies, such as the presence of nonsuperficial tumors, are not easily distinguishable from surrounding normal tissue. This makes, in some occasions, decision-making during surgery a very difficult process. During image-guided surgery, diagnostic imaging is used in conjunction with images from the operative field to improve the localization and targeting of pathologies, as well as to monitor and control treatments. The combination of tracking technologies for recording the position of the patient and the surgical instruments with preoperative and intraoperative images provides a comprehensive assistance tool for guiding any MIS intervention [27, 89–91]. Image-guided technology allows for more precise and accurate procedures, allowing surgeons to decide the best approach to address a specific disease before the intervention [92].

Radical surgical resection of tumor tissue is currently the best chance for cure. However, this option is only suitable for a minority of patients, and surgical procedures are complex with high rates of local recurrence. The presence of microscopic residual tumor tissue at the resection margins is one of the main prognostic factors, and therefore optimizing the surgical procedure to prevent positive resection margins is of the utmost importance. Accordingly, intraoperative margin assessment and visualization techniques, as well as image-guided techniques may be advantageous in guiding the surgeon to achieve curative resections.

3.1. Laparoscopic ultrasound (LUS)

Advances in technology over the last 30 years have seen the application of laparoscopic ultrasound (LUS) expand beyond its initial limited diagnostic role to assisting in tumor staging, guiding intervention, locating lesions intraoperatively, assessing anatomic relationships, and in directed therapy [93–95]. The main application of LUS during pancreatic and liver surgery is providing real-time imaging guidance for resectability assessment and detection of vessel involvement, aiming to decrease the number of irradical resections [95]. The reported overall sensitivity, specificity, and accuracy of combined diagnostic laparoscopy and LUS in predicting resectability has been reported to be 100, 91, and 96%, respectively [96]. LUS should be considered for confirmation of staging of disease when there is a strong suspicion of unresectability and tumor borders are not clearly defined by CT scan [96].

LUS plays an integral part in the management of cystic lesions of the pancreas, particularly the characterization of suspected intraductal papillary mucinous neoplasms (IPMNs) [95, 97, 98]. IPMNs appear as well-defined hypoechoic masses with associated posterior enhancement. The malignant potential of IPMNs is directly related to its relationship with the main pancreatic duct and adjacent blood vessels (**Figure 1**). LUS allows defining the cysts borders (**Figure 2**) and evaluating the relationship of the lesion with the main duct and any major vessels [95, 98, 99].

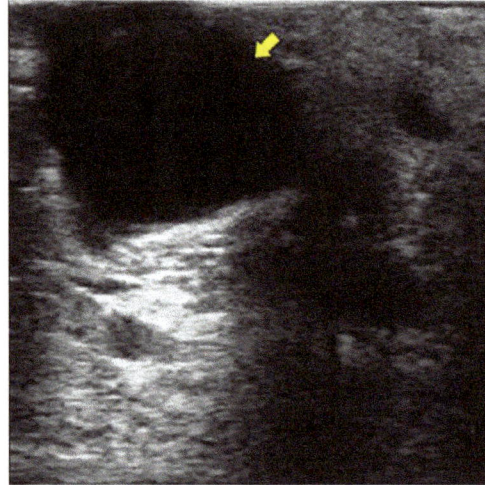

Figure 2. LUS image of a pancreatic cystic tumor. The lesion appears as a hypoechoic mass (yellow arrow).

In the case of pancreatic adenocarcinomas, they appear as a homogeneous hypoechoic mass with poorly defined margins. Large tumors can display a mixed echogenicity. A sensitivity of 90% for assessing positive lymph nodes and 100% for venous invasion have been reported for laparoscopy combined with LUS examination [100]. Regarding NETs, LUS facilitates intraoperative decision-making and demonstrates anatomic details, such as the tumor location and its relation to the adjacent vascular structures and main pancreatic duct [95, 97]. In ultrasound images, NETs typically appear as well-defined, homogeneous, and hypoechoic masses [93]. Findings from LUS inspection help to decide whether to perform either tumor enucleation or resection during laparoscopic intervention [93].

3.2. Fluorescence

Near-infrared (NIR) light (700–900 nm) is a novel imaging technique that can penetrate through several millimeters even centimeters of tissue, revealing targets below the tissue surface [101]. This imaging modality does not use ionizing radiation or direct tissue contact, making it a remarkably safe technique. NIR fluorescent contrast agents can be visualized with acquisition times in the millisecond range, enabling real-time guidance during surgery. Furthermore, as NIR light is invisible to the human eye, it does not alter the look of the surgical field, thus minimizing the learning curve [102]. The main aim of this imaging modality is to fill the gap between preoperative imaging and intraoperative reality.

Fluorescence-guided systems provide an additional tool for diagnosis of pancreatic cancer, real-time image guidance during tumor resection, and inspection to confirm complete resection [103]. This intraoperative modality can assist surgeons to visualize tumors, sentinel lymph nodes, and vital structures in real time [102]. This technology could represent the next step to improving treatment of pancreatic cancer in laparoscopic resections. However, most of the published studies for pancreatic surgery are limited to animal models.

Two main components are needed for fluorescence-guided surgery, fluorescent contrast agents and a NIR camera system. Several intraoperative NIR fluorescence camera systems have been developed for both open and laparoscopic surgery, some of which are commercially available and Food and Drug Administration (FDA) approved [104]. Fluorescent contrast agents contain a fluorescent component (fluorophore), which emits NIR fluorescent light after being excited with a NIR light source. Visualization of the tissue is based on the signal of the contrast agent in the region of interest relative to the background signal, known as signal-to-background ratio.

Indocyanine green (ICG) and methylene blue (MB) are the only NIR fluorophores that are registered with the FDA and the European Medicines Agency for clinical use. ICG emits fluorescent light at ≈800 nm and it is cleared rapidly by the liver and almost exclusively excreted into the bile, permitting imaging of bile ducts. MB has been applied clinically for many years as a visible contrast agent, and when diluted to levels that are almost undetectable to the human eye, MB becomes a fluorophore emitting at ≈700 nm. MB is cleared equally by both liver and kidney, permitting imaging of both bile ducts and ureters. ICG has been shown to accumulate around hepatic metastasis of pancreatic and colorectal cancers [105]. Methylene blue tends to accumulate in NETs after high-dose intra-arterial injection [103, 106]. The chemical structures of both ICG and MB do not allow these agents to be conjugated to tissue-specific, therefore, they are nonspecific NIR contrast agents [102, 107].

Applications of this technique during hepatopancreatobiliary surgery include tumor imaging in liver and pancreas, and real-time imaging of the biliary tree. Pessaux et al. [26] presented a robotic pancreaticoduodenectomy assisted by fluorescence imaging, providing enhanced visualization of the common bile and cystic ducts during the intervention (**Figure 1**). Subar et al. [108] reported a case of a LPD to treat an ampullary lesion in the duodenum. Before the pancreaticojejunostomy, the viability of the margin of the remnant pancreas was assessed with NIR imaging. The NIR technique improved the detection of ischemic tissue of the pancreatic margin after resection. This may lead to an increase in blood supply to the pancreatic anastomosis, and therefore potentially help to decrease the incidence of pancreatic fistulas.

In a study with different pancreatic tumors on three experimental porcine models, we analyzed the usefulness of NIR imaging during laparoscopic pancreaticoduodenectomy and single-site distal pancreatectomy procedures. In two animals, a tumor model was created in the head of the pancreas. In the third animal, the tumor model was developed in the tail of the pancreas. NIR imaging was used as guidance during LPD and LESS distal pancreatectomy. The patency of the hepaticojejunostomy was assessed by means of ICG excretion and fluoroscopic imaging. During surgery, identification of the biliary anatomy and vascular anatomy of the pancreas was possible in all procedures using NIR imaging (**Figure 3**). Biliary excretion of ICG was not clearly visualized during the patency test, but fluoroscopic imaging was positive in one case.

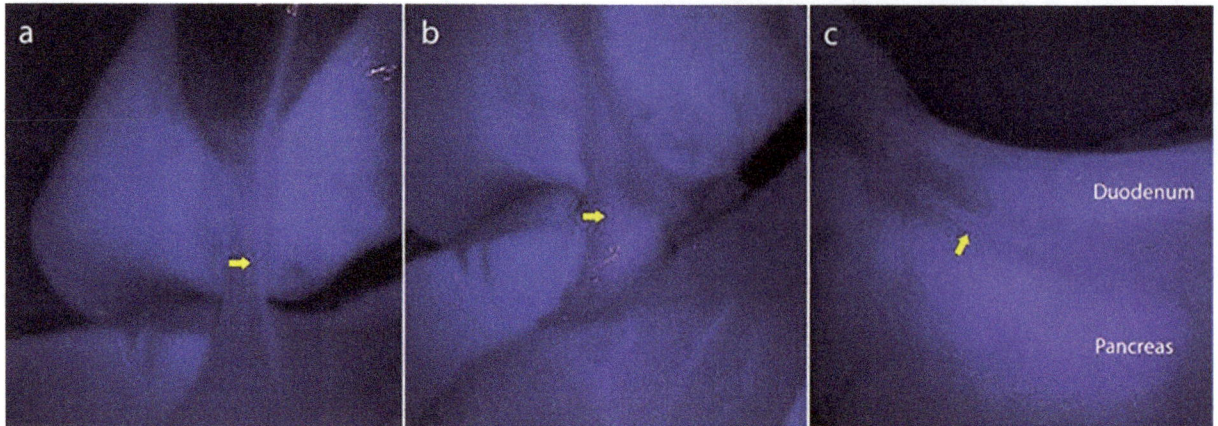

Figure 3. NIR image of biliary and pancreatic anatomy: Cystic artery (a, yellow arrow), cystic duct (b, yellow arrow), and pancreaticoduodenal artery (c, yellow arrow).

To obtain the full advantage of NIR fluorescence imaging for pancreatic cancer visualization, such as tumor imaging, tumor specific NIR conjugated agents need to be designed and tested. The tumor-targeting capability of the fluorophore-conjugated anticarcinoembryonic antigen antibody has been demonstrated in orthotopic models for intraoperative tumor visualization of both primary and metastatic deposits of pancreatic cancer [25, 109]. Metildi et al. [109] concluded that mice treated with fluorescence-guided laparoscopic surgery permitted adequate labeling and distinction of tumor margins before tumor resection, decreasing local recurrence, and increasing survival compared to mice treated with standard bright-light laparoscopic surgery.

3.3. Surgical navigation

Surgical navigation systems (SNS) combine preoperative and intraoperative image information with position and orientation tracking of surgical instruments during the surgical intervention as a surgical decision-making tool helping to improve the safety, accuracy, and efficiency of surgeries [27, 91, 92]. In MIS, due to surgeon having less visual and tactile perception compared to open surgery, image assistance becomes extensively helpful for 3D understanding of the surgical scenario and localization of lesion and essential anatomic structures.

The basic setup of a SNS consists of a preoperative image data (typically MR and CT), a tracking system (mainly electromagnetic or optical), a computer platform with screen, and the respective navigation software [89]. The combination of image-guided surgery with navigation technology consists of several steps, which are critical to ensure safety and accuracy of a procedure [27]: (1) acquisition of preoperative images and visualization for optimal diagnosis and planning, (2) accurate registration of preoperative data to the patient coordinate space and visualization in the OR, (3) intraoperative image acquisition and visualization/fusion with the preoperative images to update for anatomical shifts, and (4) postoperative imaging and visualization for evaluation of the surgical treatment.

Despite the use of navigation systems, abdominal surgery is still a challenging task. Commercial SNS are available for resection and ablation procedures of the liver (example: CAScination AG, Switzerland). However, to the best of our knowledge, no commercial systems are available or studies in the scientific literature have been published regarding the use of SNS for assistance during pancreatic cancer surgery.

We were recently able to demonstrate the usefulness of the CustusX navigation system for image guidance during a patient case, a distal pancreatectomy for the resection of a cystic tumor in the body of the pancreas (unpublished case). CustusX is an open-source navigation research platform for image-guided interventions [91]. This platform has been successfully used for many clinical applications such as neurosurgery, spine procedures, bronchoscopy, endovascular therapy, and laparoscopic procedures like adrenalectomy and lately for liver and pancreas surgery [91, 110–112].

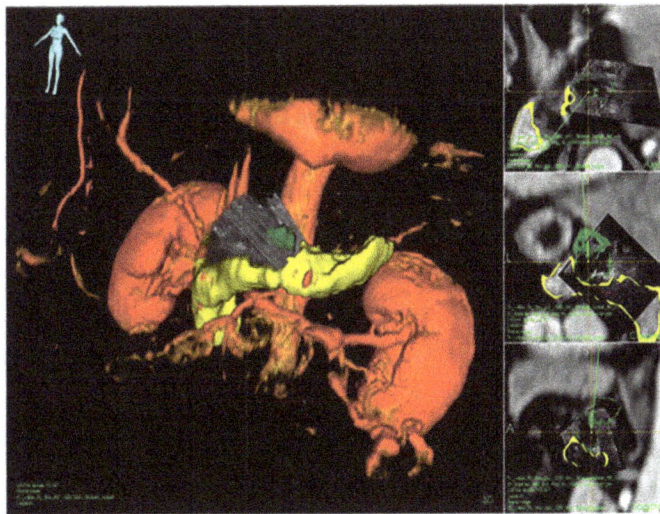

Figure 4. Snapshot of the CustusX platform during a distal pancreatectomy. The tumor is shown in green and the pancreas in yellow. The US imaging is superimposed on the 3D model from a preoperative MRI scan.

Prior to surgery, MR and CT images were acquired and imported into the navigation system software for reconstruction into 3D. The anatomical structures of interest, including the pancreas, tumor, and vessels were segmented semiautomatically [112]. The navigation system was integrated with a LUS probe running on an ultrasound scanner (Ultrasonix, Canada) with digital research interface to the navigation system. The probe was tracked by an electromagnetic sensor integrated in the tip. A probe calibration was carried out in a laboratory using a robotic arm and a well-defined geometric structure in a water tank [113]. An intraoperative registration procedure was carried out to combine the intraoperative LUS with the corresponding preoperative MR and CT images, displaying them simultaneously (**Figure 4**). This enabled the location of the lesion based on multimodal display, providing a useful tool for the surgeons to identify the anatomical structures of interest, meet their relation to other adjacent structures, and define safely and accurately the resection margin during the course of the distal pancreatectomy.

3.4. Augmented reality

Another available technology for intraoperative surgical guidance is augmented reality (AR). In surgery, AR is the fusion of artificial computer-generated images (3D virtual model) generally obtained from preoperative medical imaging and real-time patient images with the aim to visualize unapparent anatomical details. This results in the visualization of internal structures through overlying tissues, providing a virtual transparent vision of surgical anatomy. Potential advantages of the use of this imaging technology in surgery include the delineation of dissection planes or resection margins and the avoidance of injury to invisible structures.

The registration process is one of the main challenges of AR, in which the virtual model and intraoperative images should be merged in real time. In this sense, intraoperative accuracy is highly affected by mobile or deformable structures due to the heartbeat, ventilation, or laparoscopic insufflation.

A method to overlay anatomical information from preoperative CT studies onto the patient's body surface during gastrointestinal, hepatobiliary, and pancreatic surgery was presented by Sugimoto et al. [114]. For enabling the simultaneous display of the gastrointestinal tract and pancreatobiliary duct with associated blood vessels, a carbon dioxide-enhanced virtual multiple detector CT cholangiopancreatography was performed. Manual registration based on physiological markers was used. However, this method does not deal with possible alteration of the patient anatomy during the course of the surgery. A robotic pancreaticoduodenectomy assisted by AR was presented by Pessaux et al. [26]. In this study, a 3D virtual model of the patient from a preoperative CT scan was manually merged with the stereoscopic images from the da Vinci® robotic system.

4. Conclusions

Pancreatic cancer has a high mortality rate and, at the time of diagnosis, the number of patients with potentially resectable tumors is considerably low. Surgery is still the only viable option for treatment of pancreatic cancer. However, surgical procedures for pancreatic resection are complex and require high surgical expertise. Pancreatic tumors can be treated through laparoscopic surgery with similar outcomes to the conventional approach. In general, studies reported that minimally invasive pancreatic surgery is feasible, safe, and with a steep learning curve. Laparoscopic procedures reported a reduction of blood loss, length of hospital stay, and positive resection margins, as well as an improvement in spleen-preserving rates when compared to open surgery. Laparoendoscopic single-site surgery reduces the blood loss and morbidity, compared with the conventional laparoscopic approach. In robot-assisted pancreatic surgery, reported surgical outcomes are similar to laparoscopic surgery, with an apparent increase in the splenic preservation rate and negative resection margins.

Laparoscopic pancreatic surgery has some technical limitations for the surgeon such as the reduced tactile and visual information. Besides, intraoperative tumor identification may be a challenging task in some cases due to the anatomical location of the pancreas, nearby major vascular structures, and frequently inflamed surrounding pancreatic tissue. These limitations may significantly impact the surgical procedure to prevent positive resection margins. Image-guided techniques provide intraoperative margin assessment and visualization methods, which may be advantageous in guiding the surgeon to achieve curative resections, resulting in improved surgical outcomes. Reported cases of fluorescence-guided pancreatic surgery showed that this imaging technique could be beneficial in surgeries where the pancreatic anatomy is difficult to identify. Navigation systems combine preoperative and intraoperative imaging, providing location of the anatomical structures of interest with respect to surgical instruments as well as the extent of the tumor to be addressed, which allows for a safe and precise definition of resection margins. Thus, surgeons will have a comprehensive system to support and guide pancreatic surgeries, with the ultimate goal of improving surgical outcomes and increase the rate of negative resections and the subsequent positive effect on the life expectancy of the patient.

Acknowledgements

This study was supported by the Norwegian National Advisory Unit for Ultrasound and Image-Guided Therapy (St. Olav's Hospital, NTNU, SINTEF); SINTEF; St. Olavs University Hospital; Liaison Committee between the Central Norway Regional Health Authority (RHA); the Norwegian University of Science and Technology (NTNU); the Extremadura Region Government, Spain; and the European Social Fund (PO14034).

Author details

Juan A. Sánchez-Margallo[1,2], Thomas Langø[2,3*], Erlend F. Hofstad[2,3], Ronald Mårvik[3,4] and Francisco M. Sánchez-Margallo[5]

*Address all correspondence to: thomasl@sintef.no

1 Department of Medical Technology, SINTEF, Trondheim, Norway

2 Department of Computer Systems and Telematics Engineering, University of Extremadura, Badajoz, Spain

3 Norwegian National Advisory Unit on Ultrasound and Image-Guided Therapy, St. Olavs Hospital, Trondheim University Hospital, Trondheim, Norway

4 Department of Gastrointestinal Surgery, St. Olavs Hospital, Trondheim University Hospital, Trondheim, Norway

5 Jesús Usón Minimally Invasive Surgery Centre, Cáceres, Spain

References

[1] Fitzmaurice C, Dicker D, Pain A, Hamavid H, Moradi-Lakeh M, MacIntyre MF, et al. The global burden of cancer 2013. JAMA Oncol. 2015; 1(4): 505–27.

[2] Malvezzi M, Bertuccio P, Levi F, La Vecchia C, Negri E. European cancer mortality predictions for the year 2013. Ann Oncol. 2013; 24: 792–800.

[3] Siegel RL, Miller KD, Jemal A. Cancer statistics, 2015. CA Cancer J Clin. 2015; 65(1): 5–29.

[4] Howlader N, Noone AM, Krapcho M, Garshell J, Miller D, Altekruse SF, et al. SEER Cancer Statistics Review, 1975–2013. Bethesda, MD: National Cancer Institute. 2016.

[5] Ryan DP, Hong TS, Bardeesy N. Pancreatic adenocarcinoma. N Engl J Med. 2014; 371(11): 1039–49.

[6] ACS, American Cancer Society. Pancreatic Cancer. 2015. Available at: http://www.cancer.org/cancer/pancreaticcancer/detailedguide/pancreatic-cancer-pdf

[7] Eurostat. Causes of death—Deaths by country of residence and occurrence [Internet]. 2015. Available at: http://appsso.eurostat.ec.europa.eu/nui/submitViewTableAction.do

[8] Ferlay J, Steliarova-Foucher E, Lortet-Tieulent J, Rosso S, Coebergh JWW, Comber H, et al. Cancer incidence and mortality patterns in Europe: Estimates for 40 countries in 2012. Eur J Cancer. 2013; 49(6):1374–403.

[9] Harris RE. Epidemiology of pancreatic cancer. In: Harris RE, editor. Epidemiology of Chronic Disease. Burlington: Jones & Bartlett. 2013. pp. 181–90.

[10] Hamilton SR, Aaltonen LA. Tumours of the exocrine pancreas. In: Hamilton SR, Aaltonen LA, editors. World Health Organization Classification of Tumours: Pathology and Genetics of Tumours of the Digestive System. Lyon: IARC Press. 2000. pp. 219–50.

[11] Jacobs EJ, Chanock SJ, Fuchs CS, Lacroix A, McWilliams RR, Steplowski E, et al. Family history of cancer and risk of pancreatic cancer: a pooled analysis from the Pancreatic Cancer Cohort Consortium (PanScan). Int J Cancer. 2010; 127(6): 1421–8.

[12] Chen YJ, Wu SC, Chen CY, Tzou SC, Cheng TL, Huang YF, et al. Peptide-based MRI contrast agent and near-infrared fluorescent probe for intratumoral legumain detection. Biomaterials. 2014; 35: 304–15.

[13] Vincent A, Herman J, Schulick R, Hruban RH, Goggins M. Pancreatic cancer. Lancet. 2011; 378: 607–20.

[14] Hidalgo M. Pancreatic cancer. N Engl J Med. 2010; 362: 1605–17.

[15] Konstantinidis IT, Warshaw AL, Allen JN, Blaszkowsky LS, Castillo CF, Deshpande V, et al. Pancreatic ductal adenocarcinoma: is there a survival difference for R1 resections

versus locally advanced unresectable tumors? What is a "true" R0 resection? Ann Surg. 2013; 257(4):731–6.

[16]   Winter JM, Cameron JL, Campbell KA, Arnold MA, Chang DC, Coleman J, et al. 1423 pancreaticoduodenectomies for pancreatic cancer: A single-institution experience. J Gastrointest Surg. 2006; 10:1199–210.

[17]   Willett CG, Lewandrowski K, Warshaw AL, Efird J, Compton CC. Resection margins in carcinoma of the head of the pancreas. Implications for radiation therapy. Ann Surg. 1993; 217: 144–8.

[18]   Garcea G, Dennison AR, Pattenden CJ, Neal CP, Sutton CD, Berry DP. Survival following curative resection for pancreatic ductal adenocarcinoma. A systematic review of the literature. JOP. 2008; 9: 99–132.

[19]   Kato K, Yamada S, Sugimoto H, Kanazumi N, Nomoto S, Takeda S, et al. Prognostic factors for survival after extended pancreatectomy for pancreatic head cancer: influence of resection margin status on survival. Pancreas. 2009; 38(6):605–12.

[20]   Andrén-Sandberg A. Prognostic factors in pancreatic cancer. N Am J Med Sci. 2012; 4(1):9–12.

[21]   de Rooij T, Jilesen AP, Boerma D, Bonsing BA, Bosscha K, van Dam RM, et al. A nationwide comparison of laparoscopic and open distal pancreatectomy for benign and malignant disease. J Am Coll Surg. 2015; 220(3):263–70.e1

[22]   Nguyen TK, Zenati MS, Boone BA, Steve J, Hogg ME, Bartlett DL, et al. Robotic pancreaticoduodenectomy in the presence of aberrant or anomalous hepatic arterial anatomy: safety and oncologic outcomes. HPB. 2015; 17(7):594–9.

[23]   Machado MA, Surjan RC, Makdissi FF. Laparoscopic distal pancreatectomy using single-port platform: technique, safety, and feasibility in a clinical case series. J Laparoendosc Adv Surg Tech. 2015; 25(7):581–5.

[24]   Yao D, Wu S, Li Y, Chen Y, Yu X, Han J. Transumbilical single-incision laparoscopic distal pancreatectomy: preliminary experience and comparison to conventional multi-port laparoscopic surgery. BMC Surg. 2014; 14(1):105.

[25]   Cao HST, Kaushal S, Metildi CA, Menen RS, Lee C, Snyder CS, et al. Tumor-specific fluorescence antibody imaging enables accurate staging laparoscopy in an orthotopic model of pancreatic cancer. Hepatogastroenterology. 2011; 29(6):997–1003.

[26]   Pessaux P, Diana M, Soler L, Piardi T, Mutter D, Marescaux J. Robotic duodenopancreatectomy assisted with augmented reality and real-time fluorescence guidance. Surg Endosc. 2014; 28(8): 2493–8.

[27]   Langø T, Hernes TN, Mårvik R. Navigated ultrasound in laparoscopic surgery. In: Malik A, editor. Advances in Laparoscopic Surgery. Rijeka: InTech. 2012. pp. 77–98.

[28] Harrison EM, Garden OJ. Laparoscopic Ultrasound in Staging of GI Malignancies. Abdominal Ultrasound for Surgeons. New York, NY: Springer New York. 2014. pp. 129–50.

[29] Gagner M, Pomp A. Laparoscopic pylorus-preserving pancreatoduodenectomy. Surg Endosc. 1994; 8: 408e10

[30] Asbun HJ, Stauffer JA. Laparoscopic approach to distal and subtotal pancreatectomy: A clockwise technique. Surg Endosc. 2012; 25(8):2643–9.

[31] Sharpe SM, Talamonti MS, Wang CE, Prinz RA, Roggin KK, Bentrem DJ, et al. Early national experience with laparoscopic pancreaticoduodenectomy for ductal adenocarcinoma:a comparison of laparoscopic pancreaticoduodenectomy and open pancreaticoduodenectomy from the national cancer data base. J Am Coll Surg. 2015; 221(1):175–84.

[32] Abdelgadir AM, Choudhury K, Dinan MA, Reed SD, Scheri RP, Blazer DG, et al. Minimally invasive versus open pancreaticoduodenectomy for cancer: practice patterns and short-term outcomes among 7061 patients. Ann Surg. 2015; 262(2):372–7.

[33] Croome KP, Farnell MB, Que FG, Reid-Lombardo KM, Truty MJ, Nagorney DM. Total laparoscopic pancreaticoduodenectomy for pancreatic ductal adenocarcinoma: Oncologic advantages over open approaches? Ann Surg. 2014; 260(4):633–8.

[34] Kendrick ML, Cusati D.Total laparoscopic pancreaticoduodenectomy. Arch Surg. 2010; 145(1):188–93.

[35] Kim SC, Song KB, Jung YS, Kim YH, Park DH, Lee SSK, et al. Short-term clinical outcomes for 100 consecutive cases of laparoscopic pylorus-preserving pancreatoduodenectomy: improvement with surgical experience. Surg Endosc. 2013; 27(1):95–103.

[36] Machado MAC, Surjan RCT, Goldman SM, Ardengh JC, Makdissi FF. Laparoscopic pancreatic resection. From enucleation to pancreatoduodenectomy. 11-year experience. Arq Gastroenterol. 2013; 50(3):214–8.

[37] Mesleh MG, Stauffer JA, Bowers SP, Asbun HJ. Cost analysis of open and laparoscopic pancreaticoduodenectomy: A single institution comparison. Surg Endosc. 2013;27(12): 4518–23.

[38] Song KB, Kim SC, Hwang DW, Lee JH, Lee DJ, Lee JW, et al. Matched case-control analysis comparing laparoscopic and open pylorus-preserving pancreaticoduodenectomy in patients with periampullary tumors. Ann Surg. 2015; 262(1):146–55.

[39] Tran TB, Dua MM, Worhunsky DJ, Poultsides GA, Norton JA, Visser BC. The first decade of laparoscopic pancreaticoduodenectomy in the United States: costs and outcomes using the nationwide inpatient sample. Surg Endosc. 2016; 30(5):1778–83.

[40] Gagner M, Pomp A, Herrera MF. Early experience with laparoscopic resections of islet cell tumors. Surgery. 1996; 120: 1051–4.

[41] Cuschieri A, Jakimowicz JJ, van Spreeuwel J. Laparoscopic distal 70% pancreatectomy and splenectomy for chronic pancreatitis. Ann Surg. 1996; 223:280–5.

[42] Wolfgang CL, Herman JM, Laheru DA, Klein AP, Erdek MA, Fishman EK, et al. Recent progress in pancreatic cancer. CA Cancer J Clin. 2013; 63(5):318–48.

[43] Kleeff J, Diener MK, Z'graggen K, Hinz U, Wagner M, Bachmann J, et al. Distal pancreatectomy: risk factors for surgical failure in 302 consecutive cases. Ann Surg. 2007; 245(4):573–82.

[44] Lillemoe KD, Kaushal S, Cameron JL, Sohn TA, Pitt HA, Yeo CJ. Distal pancreatectomy: indications and outcomes in 235 patients. Ann Surg. 1999; 229(5): 693–8.

[45] Adam MA, Choudhury K, Goffredo P, Reed SD, Blazer D 3rd, Roman SA, et al. Minimally invasive distal pancreatectomy for cancer: short-term oncologic outcomes in 1733 patients. World J Surg. 2015; 39(10):2564–72.

[46] Braga M, Pecorelli N, Ferrari D, Balzano G, Zuliani W, Castoldi R. Results of 100 consecutive laparoscopic distal pancreatectomies: postoperative outcome, cost-benefit analysis, and quality of life assessment. Surg Endosc. 2015; 29(7):1871–8.

[47] Daouadi M, Zureikat AH, Zenati MS, Choudry H, Tsung A, Bartlett DL, et al. Robot-assisted minimally invasive distal pancreatectomy is superior to the laparoscopic technique. Ann Surg. 2013; 257(1):128–32.

[48] DiNorcia J, Schrope Ba., Lee MK, Reavey PL, Rosen SJ, Lee J a., et al. Laparoscopic distal pancreatectomy offers shorter hospital stays with fewer complications. J Gastrointest Surg. 2010; 14(11):1804–12.

[49] Gumbs AA, Croner R, Rodriguez A, Zuker N, Perrakis A, Gayet B. 200 Consecutive laparoscopic pancreatic resections performed with a robotically controlled laparoscope holder. Surg Endosc. 2013; 27(10): 3781–91.

[50] Jayaraman S, Gonen M, Brennan MF, D'Angelica MI, DeMatteo RP, Fong Y, et al. Laparoscopic distal pancreatectomy: evolution of a technique at a single institution. J Am Coll Surg. 2010; 211(4):503–9.

[51] Jean-Philippe A, Alexandre J, Christophe L, Denis C, Masson B, Fernández-Cruz L, et al. Laparoscopic spleen-preserving distal pancreatectomy. JAMA Surg. 2013; 148(3): 246–52.

[52] Kneuertz PJ, Patel SH, Chu CK, Fisher SB, Maithel SK, Sarmiento JM, et al. Laparoscopic distal pancreatectomy: Trends and lessons learned through an 11-year experience. J Am Coll Surg. 2012; 215(2):167–76.

[53] Lee SY, Allen PJ, Sadot E, D'Angelica MI, DeMatteo RP, Fong Y, et al. Distal pancreatectomy: A single institution's experience in open, laparoscopic, and robotic approaches. J Am Coll Surg. 2015; 220(1):18–27.

[54] Malleo G, Damoli I, Marchegiani G, Esposito A, Marchese T, Salvia R, et al. Laparoscopic distal pancreatectomy: Analysis of trends in surgical techniques, patient selection, and outcomes. Surg Endosc. 2015; 29(7):1952–62.

[55] Mendoza AS 3rd, Han HS, Ahn S, Yoon YS, Cho JY, Choi Y. Predictive factors associated with postoperative pancreatic fistula after laparoscopic distal pancreatectomy: A 10-year single-institution experience. Surg Endosc. 2016; 30(2): 649–56.

[56] Nakamura M, Wakabayashi G, Miyasaka Y, Tanaka M, Morikawa T, Unno M, et al. Multicenter comparative study of laparoscopic and open distal pancreatectomy using propensity score-matching. J Hepatobiliary Pancreat Sci. 2015; 22(10):731–6.

[57] Rutz DR, Squires MH, Maithel SK, Sarmiento JM, Etra JW, Perez SD, et al. Cost comparison analysis of open versus laparoscopic distal pancreatectomy. HPB. 2014; 16(10):907–14.

[58] Sahakyan MA, Kazaryan AM, Rawashdeh M, Fuks D, Shmavonyan M, Haugvik SP, et al. Laparoscopic distal pancreatectomy for pancreatic ductal adenocarcinoma: Results of a multicenter cohort study on 196 patients. Surg Endosc. 2015 [Epub ahead of print]

[59] Sharpe SM, Talamonti MS, Wang E, Bentrem DJ, Roggin KK, Prinz RA, et al. The laparoscopic approach to distal pancreatectomy for ductal adenocarcinoma results in shorter lengths of stay without compromising oncologic outcomes. Am J Surg. 2015; 209:557–563

[60] Shin SH, Kim SC, Song KB, Hwang DW, Lee JH, Lee D, et al. A Comparative Study of laparoscopic vs open distal pancreatectomy for left-sided ductal adenocarcinoma: A propensity score-matched analysis. J Am Coll Surg. 2015; 220(2):177–85.

[61] Song KB, Kim SC, Park JB, Kim YH, Jung YS, Kim MH, et al. Single-center experience of laparoscopic left pancreatic resection in 359 consecutive patients: Changing the surgical paradigm of left pancreatic resection. Surg Endosc Other Interv Tech. 2011; 25:3364–72.

[62] Stauffer JA, Rosales-Velderrain A, Goldberg RF, Bowers SP, Asbun HJ. Comparison of open with laparoscopic distal pancreatectomy: A single institution's transition over a 7-year period. HPB. 2013; 15(2):149–55.

[63] Vijan SS. Laparoscopic vs open distal pancreatectomy. Arch Surg. 2010; 145(7):616–21.

[64] Xourafas D, Tavakkoli A, Clancy TE, Ashley SW. Distal pancreatic resection for neuroendocrine tumors: Is laparoscopic really better than open? J Gastrointest Surg. 2015; 19(5):831–40.

[65] Yan J, Kuang T, Ji D, Xu X, Wang D, Zhang R, et al. Laparoscopic versus open distal pancreatectomy for benign or premalignant pancreatic neoplasms: A two-center comparative study. J Zhejiang Univ Sci B. 2015; 16(7):573–9.

[66] Yoon Y-S, Lee KH, Han H-S, Cho JY, Jang JY, Kim S-W, et al. Effects of laparoscopic versus open surgery on splenic vessel patency after spleen and splenic vessel-preserving distal pancreatectomy: A retrospective multicenter study. Surg Endosc. 2015; 29(3): 583–8.

[67] Zhou ZQ, Kim SC, Song KB, Park K-M, Lee JH, Lee Y-J. Laparoscopic spleen-preserving distal pancreatectomy: Comparative study of spleen preservation with splenic vessel resection and splenic vessel preservation. World J Surg. 2014; 38(11):2973–9.

[68] Ricci C, Casadei R, Buscemi S, Taffurelli G, D'Ambra M, Pacilio CA, et al. Laparoscopic distal pancreatectomy: What factors are related to the learning curve? Surg Today. 2015; 45(1): 50–6.

[69] Braga M, Ridolfi C, Balzano G, Castoldi R, Pecorelli N, Di Carlo V. Learning curve for laparoscopic distal pancreatectomy in a high-volume hospital. Updates Surg. 2012; 64:179–83

[70] Goyal K, Einstein D, Ibarra RA, Yao M, Kunos C, Ellis R, Brindle J, et al. Stereotactic body radiation therapy for nonresectable tumors of the pancreas. J Surg Res. 2012; 174(2): 319–25.

[71] Barbaros U, Sümer A, Demirel T, Karakullukçu N, Batman B, Içscan Y, et al. Single incision laparoscopic pancreas resection for pancreatic metastasis of renal cell carcinoma. JSLS. 2010; 14(4):566–70.

[72] Bracale U, Lazzara F, Andreuccetti J, Stabilini C, Pignata G. Single-access laparoscopic subtotal spleno-pancreatectomy for pancreatic adenocarcinoma. Minim Invasive Ther Allied Technol. 2014; 23(2):106–9.

[73] Chang SKY, Lomanto D, Mayasari M. Single-port laparoscopic spleen preserving distal pancreatectomy. Minim Invasive Surg. 2012; 2012:1–4.

[74] Han HJ, Yoon SY, Song TJ, Choi SB, Kim WB, Choi SY, Park SH. Single-port laparoscopic distal pancreatectomy: Initial experience. J Laparoendosc Adv Surg Tech A. 2014; 24(12): 858–63.

[75] Haugvik SP, Røsok BI, Waage A, Mathisen O, Edwin B. Single-incision versus conventional laparoscopic distal pancreatectomy: A single-institution case-control study. Langenbecks Arch Surg. 2013; 398:1091–6.

[76] Misawa T, Ito R, Futagawa Y, Fujiwara Y, Kitamura H, Tsutsui N, et al. Single-incision laparoscopic distal pancreatectomy with or without splenic preservation: How we do it. Asian J Endosc Surg. 2012; 5(4):195–9.

[77] Srikanth G, Shetty N, Dubey D. Single incision laparoscopic distal pancreatectomy with splenectomy for neuroendocrine tumor of the tail of pancreas. J Minim Access Surg. 2013; 9(3):132–5.

[78] Giulianotti PC, Coratti A, Angelini M, Sabrana F, Cecconi S, Balestracci T, Caravaglios G. Robotics in general surgery. Arch Surg. 2003; 138:777–84.

[79] Polanco PM, Zenati MS, Hogg ME, Shakir M, Boone BA, Bartlett DL, et al. An analysis of risk factors for pancreatic fistula after robotic pancreaticoduodenectomy: outcomes from a consecutive series of standardized pancreatic reconstructions. Surg Endosc. 2016;30(4):1523–9.

[80] Boone Ba, Zenati M, Hogg ME, Steve J, Moser AJ, Bartlett DL, et al. Assessment of quality outcomes for robotic pancreaticoduodenectomy: Identification of the learning curve. JAMA Surg. 2015; 15232(5):1–7.

[81] Hanna EM, Rozario N, Rupp C, Sindram D, Iannitti DA, Martinie JB. Robotic hepatobiliary and pancreatic surgery: Lessons learned and predictors for conversion. Int J Med Robot Comput Assist Surg. 2013; 9(2): 152–9.

[82] Shakir M, Boone Ba, Polanco PM, Zenati MS, Hogg ME, Tsung A, et al. The learning curve for robotic distal pancreatectomy: An analysis of outcomes of the first 100 consecutive cases at a high-volume pancreatic centre. HPB. 2015; 17(7): 580–6.

[83] Napoli N, Kauffmann EF, Perrone VG, Miccoli M, Brozzetti S, Boggi U. The learning curve in robotic distal pancreatectomy. Updates Surg. 2015; 67(3): 257–64.

[84] Chen S, Chen J-Z, Zhan Q, Deng X-X, Shen B-Y, Peng C-H, et al. Robot-assisted laparoscopic versus open pancreaticoduodenectomy: A prospective, matched, mid-term follow-up study. Surg Endosc. 2015; 29(12):3698–711.

[85] Giulianotti PC, Sbrana F, Bianco FM, Elli EF, Shah G, Addeo P, et al. Robot-assisted laparoscopic pancreatic surgery: Single-surgeon experience. Surg Endosc. 2010; 24(7): 1646–57.

[86] Zeh HJ, Zureikat AH, Secrest A, Dauoudi M, Bartlett D, Moser AJ. Outcomes after robot-assisted pancreaticoduodenectomy for periampullary lesions. Ann Surg Oncol. 2012; 19(3): 864–70.

[87] Zureikat AH, Moser AJ, Boone BA, Bartlett DL, Zenati M, Zeh HJ 3rd. 250 robotic pancreatic resections: Safety and feasibility. Ann Surg. 2013; 258(4):554–9.

[88] Chen S, Zhan Q, Chen J, Jin J-B, Deng X-X, Chen H, et al. Robotic approach improves spleen-preserving rate and shortens postoperative hospital stay of laparoscopic distal pancreatectomy: A matched cohort study. Surg Endosc. 2015; 29(12):3507–18.

[89] Cleary K, Wilson E, Ordas S, Banovac F. Navigation. In: Jolesz FA, editor. Intraoperative Imaging and Image-Guided Therapy. Springer, New York. 2014.

[90] Langø T, Vijayan S, Rethy A, Våpenstad C, Solberg OV, Mårvik R, et al. Navigated laparoscopic ultrasound in abdominal soft tissue surgery: Technological overview and perspectives. Int J Comput Assist Radiol Surg. 2012; 7(4):585–99.

[91] Askeland C, Solberg OV, Bakeng JBL, Reinertsen I, Tangen GA, Hofstad EF, et al. CustusX: An open-source research platform for image-guided therapy. Int J Comput Assist Radiol Surg. 2016; 11: 505–19.

[92] Sánchez-Margallo FM, Sánchez-Margallo JA. Computer-assisted minimally invasive surgery: Image-guided interventions and robotic surgery. In: Xiaojun C, editor. Computer-Assisted Surgery: New Developments, Applications and Potential Hazards. New York: Nova Science Publishers. 2015. pp. 43–95.

[93] Li W, An L, Liu R, Yao K, Hu M, Zhao G, et al. Laparoscopic ultrasound enhances diagnosis and localization of insulinoma in pancreatic head and neck for laparoscopic surgery with satisfactory postsurgical outcomes. Ultrasound Med Biol. 2011; 37(7): 1017–23.

[94] Våpenstad C, Rethy A, Langø T, Selbekk T, Ystgaard B, Hernes TAN, et al. Laparoscopic ultrasound: A survey of its current and future use, requirements, and integration with navigation technology. Surg Endosc. 2010; 24(12):2944–53.

[95] Piccolboni D, Ciccone F, Settembre a, Corcione F. Laparoscopic intra-operative ultrasound in liver and pancreas resection: Analysis of 93 cases. J Ultrasound. 2010; 13(1): 3–8.

[96] Barabino M, Santambrogio R, Pisani Ceretti A, Scalzone R, Montorsi M, Opocher E. Is there still a role for laparoscopy combined with laparoscopic ultrasonography in the staging of pancreatic cancer? Surg Endosc. 2011; 25(1):160–5.

[97] Fernández-Cruz L, Sáenz A, Astudillo E, Martinez I, Hoyos S, Pantoja JP, et al. Outcome of laparoscopic pancreatic surgery: Endocrine and nonendocrine tumors. World J Surg. 2002; 26(8):1057–65.

[98] Schachter PP, Shimonov M, Czerniak A. The role of laparoscopy and laparoscopic ultrasound in the diagnosis of cystic lesions of the pancreas. Gastrointest Endosc Clin N Am. 2002; 12(4):759–67.

[99] Schwarz L, Fleming J, Katz M, Lee J, Aloia T, Vauthey N, Conrad C. Total laparoscopic central pancreatectomy with pancreaticogastrostomy for high-risk cystic neoplasm. Ann Surg Oncol. 2016; 23(3): 1035.

[100] Catheline JM, Turner R, Rizk N, Barrat C, Champault G The use of diagnostic laparoscopy supported by laparoscopic ultrasonography in the assessment of pancreatic cancer. Surg Endosc. 1999; 13(3):239–45.

[101] Chance B. Near-infrared images using continuous, phase-modulated, and pulsed light with quantitation of blood and blood oxygenation. Ann N Y Acad Sci. 1998; 838: 29–45.

[102] Vahrmeijer AL, Hutteman M, van der Vorst JR, van de Velde CJH, Frangioni JV. Image-guided cancer surgery using near-infrared fluorescence. Nat Rev Clin Oncol. 2013; 10(9):507–18.

[103] Winer JH, Choi HS, Gibbs-Strauss SL, Ashitate Y, Colson YL, Frangioni JV. Intraoperative localization of insulinoma and normal pancreas using invisible near-infrared fluorescent light. Ann Surg Oncol. 2010; 17(4):1094–100.

[104] Chi C, Du Y, Ye J, Kou D, Qiu J, Wang J, et al. Intraoperative imaging-guided cancer surgery: From current fluorescence molecular imaging methods to future multi-modality imaging technology. Theranostics. 2014; 4(11):1072–84.

[105] Yokoyama N, Otani T, Hashidate H, Maeda C, Katada T, Sudo N. et al. Real-time detection of hepatic micrometastases from pancreatic cancer by intraoperative fluorescence imaging: Preliminary results of a prospective study. Cancer. 2012; 118:2813–9.

[106] Van der Vorst JR, Vahrmeijer AL, Hutteman M. Near-infrared fluorescence imaging of a solitary fibrous tumor of the pancreas using methylene blue. World J Gastrointest Surg. 2012; 4(7):180–4.

[107] Verbeek FPR, van der Vorst JR, Schaafsma BE, Hutteman M, Bonsing BA, van Leeuwen FWB, et al. Image-guided hepatopancreatobiliary surgery using near-infrared fluorescent light. J Hepatobiliary Pancreat Sci. 2012; 19(6):626–37.

[108] Subar D, Pietrasz D, Fuks D, Gayet B. A novel technique for reducing pancreatic fistulas after pancreaticojejunostomy. J Surg Case Rep. 2015; 2015(7): rjv074.

[109] Metildi CA, Kaushal S, Luiken GA, et al. Advantages of fluorescence-guided laparoscopic surgery of pancreatic cancer labeled with fluorescent anti-carcinoembryonic antigen antibodies in an orthotopic mouse model. J Am Coll Surg. 2014;219:132–41.

[110] Sorger H, Hofstad EF, Amundsen T, Langø T, Leira HO. A novel platform for electromagnetic navigated ultrasound bronchoscopy (EBUS). Int J Comput Assist Radiol Surg. 2015 [Epub ahead of print].

[111] Manstad-Hulaas F, Tangen GA, Dahl T, Hernes TA, Aadahl P. Three-dimensional electromagnetic navigation vs. fluoroscopy for endovascular aneurysm repair: a prospective feasibility study in patients. J Endovasc Ther. 2012; 19(1):70–8.

[112] Langø T, Tangen GA, Mårvik R, Ystgaard B, Yavuz Y, Kaspersen JH, et al. Navigation in laparoscopy-prototype research platform for improved image-guided surgery. Minim Invasive Ther Allied Technol. 2008; 17(1):17–33.

[113] Bø LE, Hofstad EF, Lindseth F, Hernes TA. Versatile robotic probe calibration for position tracking in ultrasound imaging. Phys Med Biol. 2015; 60(9): 3499–513.

[114] Sugimoto M, Yasuda H, Koda K, Suzuki M, Yamazaki M, Tezuka T, et al. Image overlay navigation by markerless surface registration in gastrointestinal, hepatobiliary and pancreatic surgery. J Hepatobiliary Pancreat Sci. 2010; 17(5):629–36.

6

Total Laparoscopic Hysterectomy

Nidhi Sharma and Vanusha Selvin

Abstract

The applications of minimally invasive pelvic surgery continue to grow. This chapter focuses primarily on the preoperative evaluation, surgical technique and post-operative care of total laparoscopic hysterectomy. Since laparoscopic assisted vaginal hysterectomy is a slight modification of the procedure it is not being discussed separately. The major physiologic obstacles to safe laparoscopy include pregnancy, increased intra cranial pressure, abnormalities of cardiac output and gaseous exchange in the lung, chronic liver diseases and coagulation disorders. In a redo surgery there may be problems of laparoscopic port entry.

Keywords: hysterectomy, laparoscopy, surgery, total laparoscopic hysterectomy, laparoscopic supracervical hysterectomy, minimally invasive gynecological procedure

1. Introduction

The invention of Veress needle by Sir Janos Veres, an internist working in Hungary on tuberculosis, launched the era of laparoscopy [1]. The first laparoscopic hysterectomy was performed by Reich in 1989 [2]. Laparoscopic hysterectomy carries an edge over open hysterectomy as it provides a better magnification of anatomy and pathology [3–6].

The three main considerations are ergonomics, task analysis and minimizing injury and adhesions. When we apply the baseball diamond concept of trocar placement, the target in total laparoscopic hysterectomy is the uterine artery.

2. Preoperative evaluation

The goal of preoperative evaluation is to identify and modify risk factors that might adversely affect anesthetic care and surgical outcome.

2.1. History

1. Pulmonary disease—either obstructive or restrictive lung disease.
2. Cardiac disease
3. History of previous abdominal surgeries
4. History of coagulation disorders in self or in family
5. Previous history of anesthesia related complications
6. History of dentures or prosthetic devices
7. Previous operative records if any

2.2. Physical examination

1. Assessment of head and neck
2. Assessment of lungs and heart
3. Vascular and neurological examination
4. Airway evaluation by anesthetist
5. Vital signs
6. Abdominal examination to look for scar site and to decide on alternate port site and to assess the extent of adhesions.

2.3. Basic prerequisites before laparoscopic surgery

1. Hemoglobin
2. Blood urea and creatinine
3. Serum electrolytes
4. Liver function test
5. Coagulation profile
6. ECG and chest X-ray
7. Serology testing
8. Ultrasound abdomen and pelvis
9. Urine analysis

Tests obtained within 6 months of surgery are acceptable if there is no significant change in patient medical history.

2.4. Patient education

The expectations with regard to the surgery should be clearly discussed with the patient. Anesthetic and surgical procedure and complications should be clearly explained to the patient. Risk of perioperative morbidity and mortality, post op pain, recovery, length of stay everything in detail should be counseled to the patient prior to surgery. Detailed informed consent regarding chance of conversion to laparotomy, chance of visceral injury should be obtained.

3. Surgical technique

The laparoscopic hysterectomy is classified depending on the extent of dissection done laparoscopically (**Table 1**). The knowledge of anatomy is essential before hysterectomy (**Figure 1**). The sterile precautions are maintained to arrange and assemble the laparoscopy instruments (**Figure 2**).

3.1. Positioning

The patient is given general anesthesia, with oral tracheal intubation. The patient is positioned in dorsal decubitus position Loyd Davis Position. The legs are positioned in the low lithotomy position with thighs flexed at 30°and knees supported, the arms are positioned along the body, and the buttocks extending slightly over the edge of the surgical table. The bladder is catheterized. The surgeon is positioned to the left of the patient. The first assistant

Hysterectomy Type	Description
I	Diagnostic laparoscopy and vaginal hysterectomy
II	Laparoscopic assisted vaginal Hysterectomy
III	Laparoscopic hysterectomy
IV	Total Laparoscopic Hysterectomy
V	Laparoscopic supracervical Hysterectomy
VI	Vaginal Hysterectomy with Laparoscopic Vault suspension
VII	Laparoscopic Hysterectomy with lymphadenectomy
VIII	Laparoscopic hysterectomy with lymphadenectomy and omentectomy
IX	Laparoscopic radical hysterectomy and lymphadenectomy

Table 1. The classification of laparoscopy assisted hysterectomy.

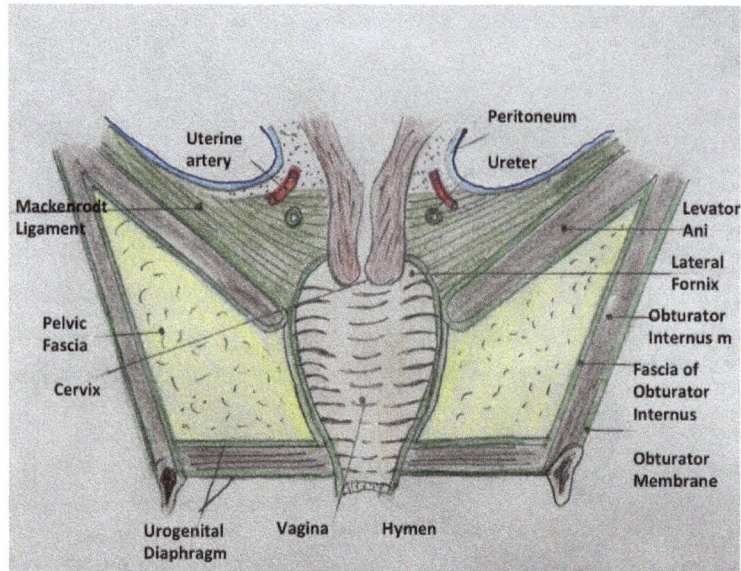

Figure 1. A sagittal section of a cadaveric specimen of female pelvis showing the anterior and posterior relation of the uterus.

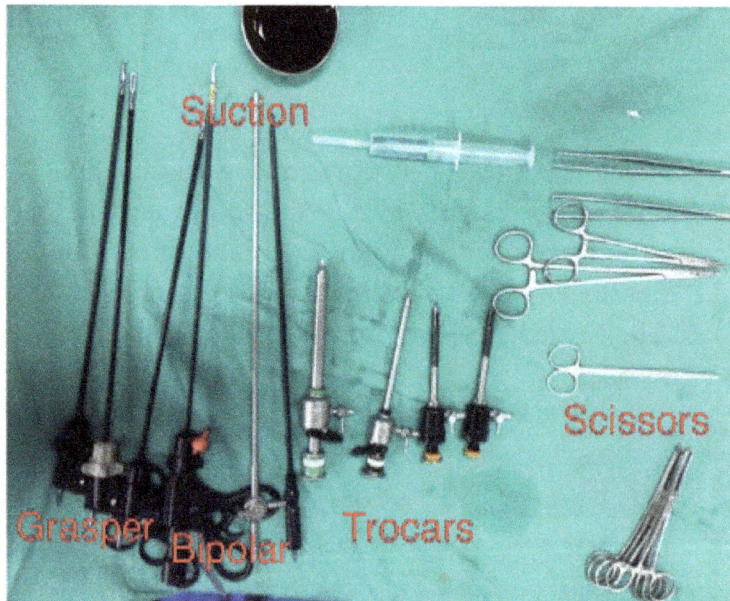

Figure 2. The laparoscopy instruments required are arranged in a sterile cart: grasper, bipolar, scissors, suction irrigation, trocars and cannula. One 10 mm and three 5 mm ports are necessary.

is on the right side of the patient. The second assistant does the uterine manipulation and he stands between the legs of the patient. A foam mattress is placed directly under the patient to prevent sliding during steep Trendelenburg. The table is kept in a low position to enable wrist movements for intracorporeal knotting. The monitor to directly face each surgeon at the angle of resting eye, i.e., 30°, to promote an ergonomic working environment. The surgeon, the target tissue and the monitor should be in straight line. The height of the table should be about the half of surgeons' height to enable wrist movements.

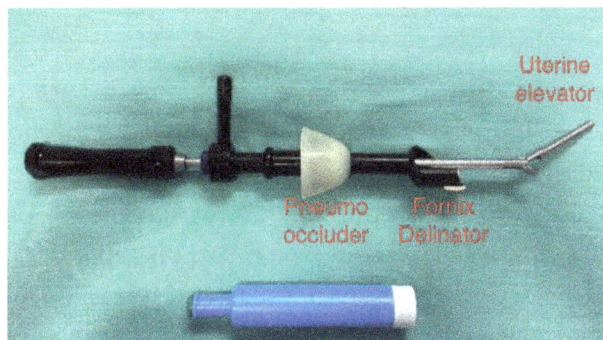

Figure 3. The uterine manipulator is used to antevert the uterus and delineate the fornixes for laparoscopic colpotomy. The pneumoperitoneum is maintained by the soft silastic parts of the instrument that prevent the air leak after colpotomy.

3.2. Vaginal manipulation

Uterine cannulation is performed with a specific instrument named The Clermont-Ferrand type Karl Storz Uterine Manipulator or RUMI - Uterine Manipulator (**Figure 3**).

First, a Sims speculum is placed into the vagina. Cervix is held with a tenaculum and the uterus is sounded. The cervix is dilated to Hegar number 9. RUMI tip used should be selected according to the patient after sounding the uterine cavity with a uterine sound. If the uterine cavity is 7, a 6-cm tip should be selected. The sizes available are 6, 8, or 10 cm. The distal end of the shaft may be dipped in the in lubricant prior to attaching the tip. This greatly facilitates the insertion into the uterine cavity. The pneumo-occluder is now slid over the tip and the shaft. Now the Koh cup (3, 3.5, and 4 cm in width) is attached. The Koh cup should be appropriately sized according to the cervix of the patient. This is important because a small ring will not mark the vaginal fornices exactly and only push up the cervix. The delineation of fornices is important because it serves as a landmark till the surgery is complete. A large ring will increase the risk of a ureteral injury. Insert the tip of the RUMI as far into the cervix as it will go. The correct placement is confirmed by palpation or direct visualization. Inflate the Uterine balloon with 5 cc of normal saline to manipulate the uterus and facilitate specimen removal through the vagina at the end of the case. The bladder is catheterized with Foleys catheter. The pneumo-occluder is now inflated with 60 to 100 cc of saline. RUMI II and RUMI arc are recent modifications that fasciate easy manipulation.

3.3. Establishing the pneumo-peritoneum

The stomach should be deflated by Ryle's tube insertion and aspiration. First step is to insert the Veress needle following the double click sound at subumbilical incision or the Palmer's point in the left upper quadrant, about 2 to 3 cm below the left costal margin, in the left mid-clavicular line [7]. Now, CO_2 insufflation is done to create pneumoperitoneum to achieve an intra-abdominal pressure of 12 to 14 mmHg [8, 9]. An easy way to confirm intraperitoneal entry is to look for the pressure reading on the insufflator. If the pressure reading is high the Veress needle is likely to be impinging on the omentum. A slight gentle movement will dislodge it. Alternatively bubble test can be done.

3.4. Positioning the trocar

Four trocars are positioned: one 10 mm umbilical trocar with a 30° optic and three 5 mm trocars, with one 2 cm medial to the right superior iliac crest, another 2 cm medial to the left anterior superior iliac crest, and a third in the midline, 8–10 cm below the umbilical port. These trocars are placed lateral to the rectus abdominis muscles, 2 cm above and 2 cm medial to the anterior superior iliac spine (**Figure 4**). The last 5 mm trocar can be substituted by a 10–15 mm trocar during surgery for the introduction of suture needles and for suturing of the vaginal vault. A complete survey of the abdomen to rule out any visceral injury at the time of entry is done. The lower quadrant trocar sleeves are placed under direct vision. In the case of very voluminous uteri, the trocars can be positioned more cephalad using the diamond baseball concept.

3.5. Visualization of pelvic organs

After inserting the ports the trocars are withdrawn and instruments are inserted. The patient is placed in 15° head low position to move the bowel loops away from pelvis. The small intestine loops are mobilized upwards to visualize the uterus, tubes, ovaries, round ligaments and infundibulopelvic ligaments. The surgeon uses a grasper and a bipolar and follows the manipulation angle of 60°. The Azimuth angle is maintained at 30°. Manipulation angle is the angle between the two operating instruments. Azimuth angle is the angle between the scope and the operating instrument. The first assistant holds the scope with the left hand and uses the Maryland grasper forceps in the right hand. If adhesions are seen they should be gently released. Releasing adhesions between sigmoid colon and utero-ovarian ligament permits the correct exposure of the infundibulopelvic ligament and posterior surface of the uterus. The sequence to be followed is look, hook, coagulate and cut. Thick tissue should be cauterized in small steps with coagulating cautery set at 35 W to prevent charring. The uterus is mobilized by the second assistant and is maintained cranially and anteriorly.

3.6. Coagulation and section of round ligament

The round ligament is secured with traction by the first assistant, making possible its exposure for the start of the surgery. The round ligament is coagulated at a distance of 2 to 3 cm from the lateral pelvic wall using a bipolar cautery (**Figure 5**). The coagulation of the round

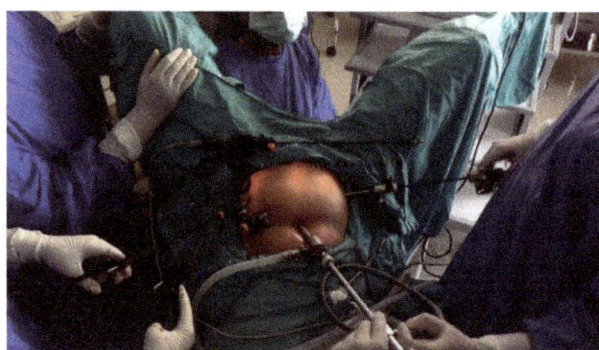

Figure 4. Laparoscopic port positions for total laparoscopic hysterectomy with ipsilateral pports. The infraumbilical port is the telescopic port. The right iliac fossa port is the traction port and the two left iliac fossa ports are the operating ports.

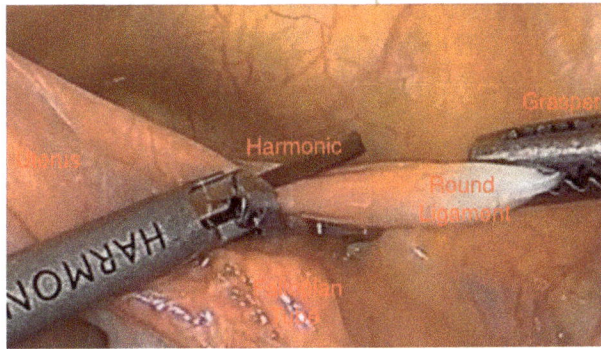

Figure 5. The round ligament is held 2–3 cm from the lateral pelvic wall. The ligament is coagulated with bipolar and cut with scissors.

ligament near the uterus is difficult as there is an artery to the round ligament which may bleed. This is followed by opening the anterior leaflet of the broad ligament to the vesico-uterine peritoneal reflection.

3.7. Coagulation and section of the infundibulo-pelvic ligament

The first assistant should secure the adnexa and apply traction in a direction opposite to the operating side (**Figure 6**). The coagulation and sectioning of the ligament should be progressive, plane to plane (peritoneum, followed by the vessels and connective tissue). The infundibulopelvic ligament or the tubo-ovarian ligament are now coagulated and with a bipolar grasper and scissors. The infundibulopelvic ligament should be coagulated close to the ovary (hug the ovary) as this helps to avoid injury to the vital structures in the pelvic sidewall. The tubo-ovarian ligament should also be coagulated close to the ovary to prevent injury to the uterine vessel during ovarian conservation. When you want to preserve the adnexa, the coagulation and section is performed proximal to the fallopian tubes and the utero-ovarian ligament. The posterior leaf of broad ligament is opened with incision extending till the internal os being careful not to injure the uterine artery and vein (**Figure 7**). The peritoneum is opened, coagulated and cut till the attachment of the utero-sacral ligaments. The capillaries in the posterior leaf of broad ligament and the parametrial veins that run between the ovary and round ligament should be taken care of.

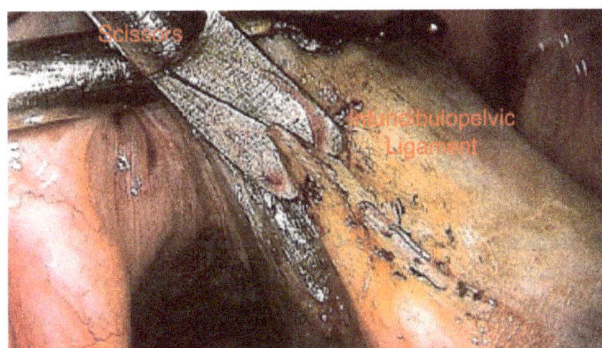

Figure 6. The infundibulopelvic ligament is identified by gentle traction. It is also coagulated with bipolar and cut with scissors.

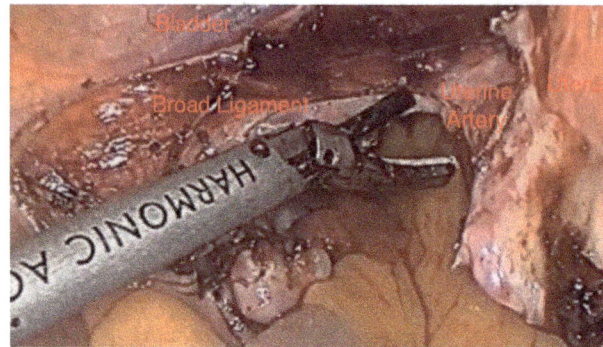

Figure 7. The peritoneum in the broad ligament is opened and uterine vessels are identified at the level of internal os.

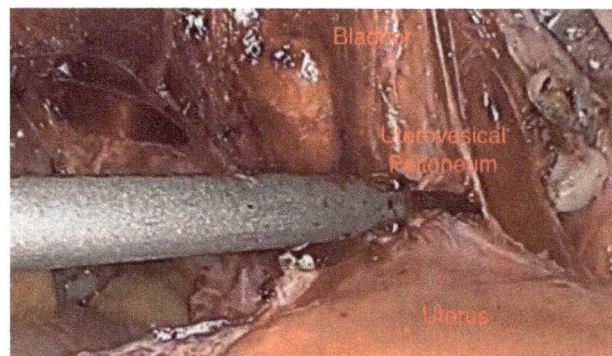

Figure 8. The loose vesicouterine fold of peritoneum is held with grasper and scissors used to dissect the bladder. The bladder is gently dissected downwards by laparoscopic pledgets or applying traction from the jaws of bipolar.

3.8. Mobilization of bladder

The assistant uses an atraumatic forceps to grasp the peritoneum and the bladder in the midline, applying vertical and cranial traction (**Figure 8**). The peritoneum and the adjacent connective tissue are coagulated and sectioned, thus accessing the vesico-vaginal plane and posteriorly to expose the bottom of vesico-uterine sac. The dissection continues in a caudal direction, initially in the midline and then laterally, performing the coagulation and section of the vesico-uterine ligaments thereby mobilizing the bladder off the lower uterine segment. The plane of loose areolar tissue should be identified and opened avoiding injury to the vessels. In women with previous cesarean delivery, there are adhesions between bladder and lower uterine surface and so dissection should be a little high as close to the uterus as possible to avoid bladder injury.it is important to identify and pick small bits of tissue close to the uterus and coagulate and cut them gradually moving down towards the cervix [10]. Alternatively a lateral approach of opening the broad ligament may be the preferred route [11, 12]. During laparoscopic hysterectomy, if the patient has significant adhesions from prior cesarean deliveries, a reverse inferior to superior vesico-uterine fold dissection can be used to dissect the bladder from the uterus [13]. This lateral dissection and accessing the bladder from below can be used as an alternative to the commonly practiced technique of mobilizing the bladder in a superior to inferior fashion at the time of laparoscopic hysterectomy. The anatomy of the space of Seth can be helpful in identifying the lateral structures of bladder. Space of Seth is bounded laterally by the tangential line joining the maximum bulging on the uterine body and cervix, medially the bladder comes in contact with the uterocervical surface thickening at the level of bladder pillars. Anteriorly there is the undersurface of bladder and anterior leaf of broad ligament, posteriorly there is the uterocervical surface [14].

A reevaluation of the route of dissection is advised if fat is encountered because the fat belongs to the bladder and this may indicate that the dissection is moving too close to the bladder. With this the ureter is kept out-of-the-way, since it is mobilized along with the peritoneum.

3.9. Secure uterine vessels

Desiccate the ascending uterine vessels with the bipolar grasper at the level of internal cervical os. The RUMI uterine can be pushed upwards to increase the distance between uterine artery and. The uterine vessels should coagulate till there is vaporization and bubble formation. The uterine vessels should be grasped perpendicularly to coagulate the 7 mm lumen efficiently. If the uterine are grasped obliquely the lumen to be coagulated becomes wider. Grasping the uterine artery perpendicularly is made easier by the new articulating instruments which can change direction and allow the uterine artery to be grasped and coagulated perpendicularly (**Figure 9**). After the coagulation and cutting of uterine arteries the vascular pedicles are deflected laterally and dissection is continued in the avascular plane over the cervix towards the delineated vaginal fornices (**Figure 10**). The ureters should be reconfirmed and the dissection continued close to the uterus [15].

3.10. Removal of uterus

While pushing cephalad with the uterine manipulator, vaginal fornices are identified. It is identified by indentation of the Rumi Koh colpotomizer or by palpation with a laparoscopic instrument. The Harmonic scalpel or laparoscopic monopolar hook is then used to cut circumferentially around the cup, thus uterus with cervix is separated from vaginal apex (**Figures 11 and 12**). In patients with limited vaginal access, the uterus can be morcellated using an electronic morcellator and specimen removed abdominally. It is important to keep the tip of the morcellator in clear view at all times.

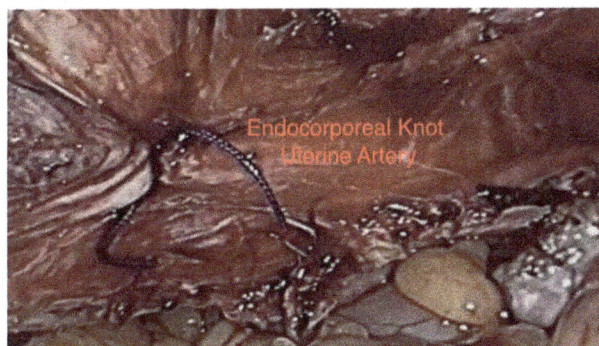

Figure 9. The uterine vessels are secured with endocorporeal knotting or harmonic.

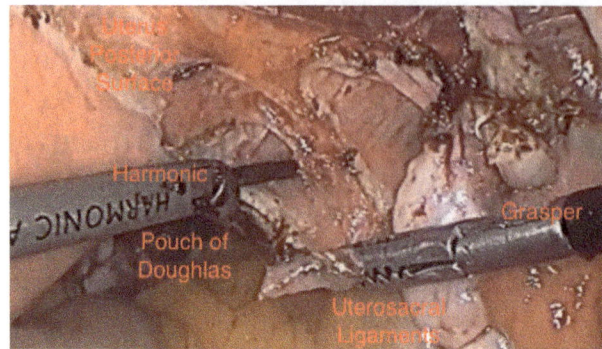

Figure 10. Uterosacral ligaments are identified and the peritoneal incision is extended to the pouch of douglas. The peritoneal incision is above the uterosacral ligaments.

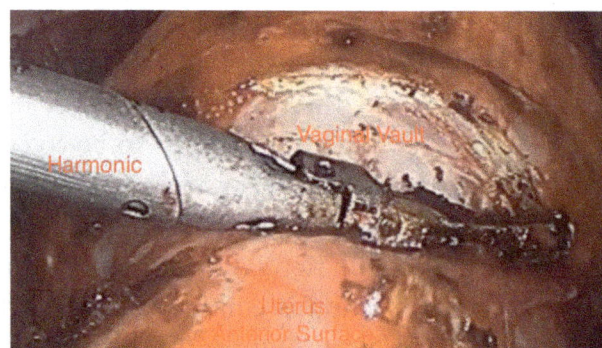

Figure 11. The vaginal vault is incised with a harmonic or laparoscopy monopolar hook after delineating the fornixes. The vaginal vault is incised above the attachment of uterosacral ligaments.

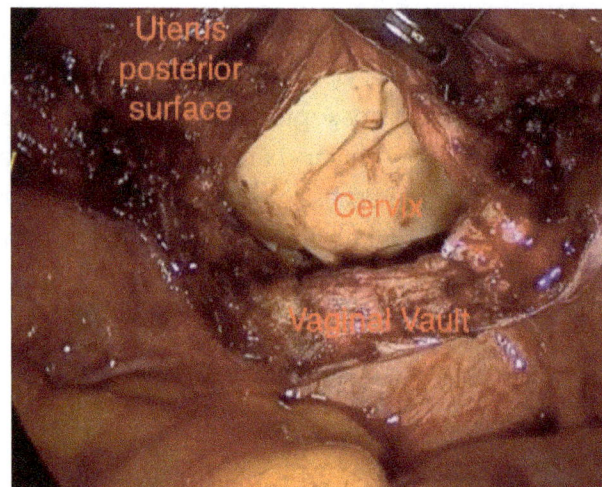

Figure 12. The posterior lip of cervix is seen after vaginal vault is incised. The pneumoperitoneum leakage is prevented by the RUMI manipulator in the vagina.

3.11. Vaginal cuff closure

Vaginal cuff should closed beginning at the margins of angle of the vaginal canal. The barb sutures are continued in running manner. The vaginal mucosa and the pubocervical and recto-vaginal fascia are included in the suture line. Each suture should be placed at 1 cm in distance from vaginal cuff margins. This is important and can be guessed as a comparison to the wide open jaw of grasper which is 2 cm wide. Distances can be easily underestimated because of the magnification of the laparoscope. Irrigation and suction is performed and hemostasis rechecked. The bidirectional barbed suture is available in which wound tension is evenly distributed across the length of the suture line rather than at the knotted end. No knots are required with bidirectional barbed suture. Since uterosacral ligament attachment to vagina is undisturbed in Total Laparoscopic hysterectomy the vaginal vault fixation is not required.

No routine cystoscopy is needed to ensure ureteral patency and bladder injury except in cases of dense bladder adhesions. However cystoscopy does not identify delayed thermal injury to ureters and bladder.

The pneumoperitoneum is deflated.

3.12. Port wound closure

The fascial defect of the 10 mm trocar in the midline is sutured and the skin is sutured with 3–0 monofilament absorbable suture.

Laparoscopic direct visualization fascial closure methods provide more accurate placement of sutures under direct vision.

Recommendations regarding port wound closure:

1. All ports greater than 10 mm either in midline or lateral should be closed at fascial level.

2. 5 mm ports if manipulated extensively or enlarged significantly during the procedure need to be closed

3. Port closure should include fascia and peritoneum.

The LigaSure Vessel Sealer, The EnSeal—Advanced Tissue Sealing Technology and the Ultracision ® harmonic scalpel are newer advances in laparoscopic surgery. Articulating vessel sealer helps to grasp and coagulate the vessel at right angle to the course of the vessel, thereby minimizing the diameter of vessel to be coagulated. Each surgeon should develop his own routine and use the available materials and technology to facilitate the surgical procedure.

4. Advantages of laparoscopic hysterectomy

1. Small surgical wound

2. Short hospital stay

3. Quick recovery

4. No abdominal wound

5. Decrease in intra op bleeding

6. Decrease in post op pain and infection

7. Low incidence of DVT.

8. Early return of bowel activity

9. Less risk of adhesion formation

5. Indications for conversion to open procedure

5.1. Planned conversion

1. Failure to progress

2. Dense or extensive lower abdominal or pelvic adhesions

3. Acute or chronic inflammatory changes causing increased vascularity resulting in tethering or tearing of tissues.

4. Difficulty to maintain pneumoperitoneum due to gas leaks in and around the ports.

5. Poor or inadequate exposure—obesity may preclude placement of ports

6. Altered or aberrant or unclear anatomy

7. Inexperience of the surgeon

5.2. Emergency conversion

1. Technical problem/instrument malfunction

2. Anesthesia related issues like—poorly tolerating pneumoperitoneum

3. Complex viscus injury

The surgeon should keep in mind the time of dissection and the progress made as well as the remaining tasks to be completed. Also the surgeon's threshold for conversion should be low while gaining experience.

6. Adhesion prevention during laparoscopic surgery

1. Minimize tissue damage

2. Perfect hemostasis

3. Minimize length of insufflation

4. Minimize intra-abdominal pressure

5. Adequate irrigation to avoid desiccation

6. Gentle tissue manipulation

7. Physical barriers like Seprafilm/Intercede

7. Post-operative pain management

There is a documented reduction in the narcotic requirement after laparoscopic Hysterectomy when compared to open procedure. It is also associated with earlier return of bowel function, earlier discharge, and improved pulmonary function.

Post op pain is due to irritation of somatic nerve fibers by overdistension of the diaphragm and carbon dioxide pneumoperitoneum related acidic intraperitoneal environment. Peritoneal ischemia, distension neurapraxia are other mechanisms that account for post op pain.

Method of reducing postoperative pain:

1. Infiltration of abdominal wall incision with local anesthetics

2. Intra peritoneal instillation of saline at the end of the procedure

3. Epidural analgesia

4. Complete removal of insufflated gas

5. Postoperative non-steroidal anti-inflammatory drugs

7.1. Prophylaxis against deep vein thrombosis

The addition of deep vein thrombosis prophylaxis should be at the discretion of the operating surgeon based upon the earlier recommendations and risk assessment of that particular patient.

7.2. Prevention of post-operative wound infection

1. Optimize the patient and iatrogenic risk factors.

2. Appropriate use of systemic perioperative antibiotics.

3. Adequate operative site preparation.

4. Avoid unnecessary trauma from hair removal techniques.

5. Avoid wiping off antiseptic after the skin preparation

6. Strict adherence to principles of sterility

7. Wide preparation of skin in case of conversion to laparotomy.

8. Adequate sized skin incisions will prevent ischemia and marginal wound necrosis.

9. Occlusive dressings to be released after 48 h because they might be conducive to bacterial overgrowth.

How to avoid Port site bleeding complications?

1. The trocar and the port should enter the abdomen at 90° to skin surface.

2. Dermal incision should be complete before using the trocar to penetrate the fascia.

3. Surgeon should be familiar with the mechanics of the given trocar.

4. Port placement should be made either in the midline or lateral to the edge of rectus sheath to avoid inferior epigastric artery.

5. Blunt tip ports are preferable to sharp tipped ones.

7.3. Post-operative advice

1. Advice to start on liquids after 6 h and to a regular light diet as tolerated on first day.

2. Bath after 48 h—for skin incision to re-epithelialize.

3. No restriction to walking from first post op day.

4. Resumption to preoperative activity by second week.

5. Regular exercise encouraged after 4 weeks.

6. Resumption of driving depends on mobility, reaction time, patient ability to respond to any road hazard. Usually resumes by 1–2 weeks.

7. Return to work by 2 weeks.

8. Continue Hematinics and Calcium supplements for 3 months.

9. Abstinence for 6 weeks.

7.4. How to avoid port site hernia

1. Minimum number of ports with smallest possible diameter.

2. Violent torqueing of port which can enlarge fascial defect.

3. Slow desufflation of abdomen while removing the ports—rapid removal of ports may draw bowel and omentum into port sites.

4. Before closure of ports shake the abdomen to dislodge the stuck bowel.

5. Closure of fascial defects before patient is extubated.

7.5. Port site seroma

It is a painless ballotable swelling at a healing port site. It usually occurs within 1–5 days post-operatively. There is no evidence of inflammation. It usually resolves spontaneously within days unless complicated by secondary bacterial infection.

7.6. Port site tumors

Port site tumor is common when an unexpected malignant specimen is retrieved through one of the ports. Serious complication has been noted in setting of ovarian cancer and to lesser extent in patients with endometrial cancer and rare in cervical cancer patients. The presence of 10–15 mm Hg pneumoperitoneum may facilitate the dispersion of liberated tumor cells throughout the abdomen and to port site during insufflation events. The employment of specimen bags is recommended to retrieve the specimen. Laparoscopic skill level of the surgeon also plays a critical factor.

8. Conclusion

Laparoscopy offers the advantage of clear magnified anatomy and pathology. The adhesions can be dissected carefully under vision. To minimize complications the basic principles that should be kept in mind can be summarized.

1. Proper patient selection

2. Adequate experience of the surgeon and assistants

3. Proper port placement

4. Avoid gas leaks

5. Sound surgical techniques

6. Adequate sized incisions

7. Thorough irrigation of port and abdomen before closure

8. Fascial and peritoneal wound closure for 10 mm or larger ports

Acknowledgements

Authors thank the nursing staff of Department of Obstetrics and Gynecology, Department of Radiology and Department of Anesthesiology, Saveetha Medical College, Chennai, for the care given to the women. We also thank the staff of Operation theaters and staff of blood bank. We thank the Biotechnical Department of Saveetha Medical College and hospital.

We also acknowledge the funds provided by Saveetha University, Chennai for the laparoscopy surgical care for women.

Conflict of interest

The authors declare that there is no conflict of interest.

Author details

Nidhi Sharma* and Vanusha Selvin

*Address all correspondence to: drbonuramkumar@yahoo.co.in

Saveetha Medical College, Saveetha University, Chennai, India

References

[1] Veres J. Neues instrument zur ausfuhrung von brust-oder bauchpunktionen und pneu-mothoraxbehandlung. Deutsche Medizinische Wochenschrift. 1938;**64**:1480-1481

[2] Reich H, DeCaprio J, McGlynn F. Laparoscopic hysterectomy. Journal of Gynecologic Surgery. 1989;**5**:213-216

[3] Reich H. Laparoscopic hysterectomy. Surgical Laparoscopy and Endoscopy. 1992;**2**:85-88

[4] Liu CY. Laparoscopic hysterectomy: A review of 72 cases. The Journal of Reproductive Medicine. 1992;**37**:351-354

[5] Liu CY. Laparoscopic hysterectomy. Report of 215 cases. Gynaecological Endoscopy. 1992;**1**:73-77

[6] Reich H, McGlynn F, Sekel L. Total laparoscopic hysterectomy. Gynaecological Endoscopy. 1993;**2**:59-63

[7] Palmer R. Instrumentation et technique de la coelioscopie gynecologique. Gynecologie Et Obstetrique (Paris). 1947;**46**:420-431. PMID 18917806

[8] Gould JC, Philip A. Principles and techniques of abdominal access and physiology of pneumoperitoneum. Scientific American Surgery. 2011;**8**:P1-P9

[9] Molloy D, Kaloo PD, Cooper M, et al. Laparoscopic entry: A literature review and analysis of techniques and complications of primary port entry. The Australian & New Zealand Journal of Obstetrics & Gynaecology. 2002;**42**:246-253

[10] Wang L, Merkur H, Hardas G, Soo S, Lujic S. Laparoscopic hysterectomy in the presence of previous caesarean section: A review of one hundred forty-one cases in the Sydney west advanced pelvic surgery unit. Journal of Minimally Invasive Gynecology. 2010;**17**(2):186-191. DOI: 10.1016/j.jmig.2009.11.007

[11] Sinha R, Sundaram M, Lakhotia S, Hedge A, Kadam P. Total laparoscopic hysterectomy in women with previous cesarean sections. Journal of Minimally Invasive Gynecology. 2010;**17**(4):513-517. DOI: 10.1016/j.jmig.2010.03.018. PMID: 20621012

[12] Celle C, Pomés C, Durruty G, Zamboni M, Cuello M. Total laparoscopic hysterectomy with previous cesarean section using a standardized technique: Experience of Pontificia Universidad Catolica de Chile. Gynecological Surgery. 2015;**12**(3):149-155

[13] Nezhat C, Grace LA, Razavi GM, Mihailide C, Bamford H. Reverse vesicouterine fold dissection for laparoscopic hysterectomy after prior cesarean deliveries. Obstetrics and Gynecology. 2016;**128**(3):629-633. DOI: 10.1097/AOG.0000000000001593. PMID: 27500328

[14] Sheth SS. Reverse vesicouterine fold dissection for laparoscopic hysterectomy after prior cesarean deliveries. Obstetrics & Gynecology. 2017;**129**(4):749-750. DOI: 10.1097/AOG.0000000000001954

[15] Manoucheri E, Cohen SL, Sandberg EM, Kibel AS, Einarsson J. Ureteral injury in laparoscopic gynecologic surgery. Reviews in Obstetrics and Gynaecology. 2012;**5**(2):106-111

7

Bariatric and Metabolic Surgery

Chih Kun Huang, Sir Emmanuel S. Astudillo,

Prasad M. Bhukebag and Khan Wei Chan

Abstract

Obesity as a global epidemic has rapidly increased in incidence in the recent few decades and represents one of the biggest public health challenges. Obesity plays a major risk for various diseases such as cardiovascular disease (CVD), diabetes mellitus (DM), hyper-cholesterolemia, osteoarthritis and some form of cancers. Bariatric and metabolic surgery provides the best solution for obesity and its associated comorbidities. This chapter will discuss in detail the commonly performed bariatric and metabolic surgeries.

Keywords: bariatric surgery, metabolic surgery, Roux-en-Y gastric bypass, sleeve gastrectomy, duodenojejunal bypass, proximal jejunal bypass, obesity, type 2 diabetes

1. Introduction

Bariatric surgery has been established to be the most effective treatment for morbid obesity, producing sustained and durable weight loss with improvement or remission of comorbidities and longer life [1]. The procedures undertaken to treat morbid obesity have changed over a period of time and recently newer procedures are being developed with lesser morbidity and mortality and better results. The resolution of comorbidities such as type 2 diabetes mellitus (T2DM), hypertension and others after bariatric surgery gave impetus to the concept of metabolic surgery. Metabolic surgery has become increasingly effective and accepted option for patients with T2DM [2]. This chapter will describe in detail two most commonly performed procedures, laparoscopic sleeve gastrectomy (LSG) and laparoscopic Roux-en-Y gastric bypass (LRYGB). Part of the chapter also details the sleeve gastrectomy-based procedures which include sleeve gastrectomy with loop duodenojejunal bypass (LDJB-SG) and sleeve gastrectomy with proximal jejunal bypass (SG-PJB).

2. Laparoscopic sleeve gastrectomy

Laparoscopic Sleeve Gastrectomy (LSG) or "sleeve" is now one of the most commonly performed bariatric procedures worldwide. It is a purely restrictive procedure without intestinal bypass. In 1999, Michel Gagner and his team performed the first laparoscopic duodenal switch on the porcine model and found it to be feasible. Laparoscopic duodenal switch was later performed in morbid obese patients and found to have higher morbidity in higher BMI patients. Staged procedure was then undertaken to reduce the mortality and morbidity with laparoscopic sleeve gastrectomy as the first stage of a two-stage duodenal switch. However, the initial weight loss after LSG alone was found to be adequate and maintained over a period of time. The second stage of surgery was deferred or was not required at all and patients maintained good weight loss with just the first stage. After this success and some modifications to the procedure, sleeve gastrectomy was established as an effective stand-alone bariatric procedure.

Apart from restriction of size of stomach, reduction in the "hunger hormone" ghrelin, after LSG decreases appetite. Advantages of LSG include lower operative complexity, relative safety and maintenance of pylorus and easy convertibility to other procedures. Also, since there are no bowel bypass problems of internal herniation, small bowel obstruction, micronutrient deficiencies and malnutrition will not be encountered.

The disadvantages of the procedure include irreversibility, possibility of staple line leak, bleeding and stricture of gastric tube. The incidence of gastroesophageal reflux has also been found to be increased in some patients undergoing this procedure.

2.1. Indications and contraindications

Indications for this procedure include BMI ≥ 40 kg/m^2 without comorbidities or ≥ 35 kg/m^2 with comorbidities. This can also be offered as a first stage of biliopancreatic diversion in patients with BMI > 50 kg/m^2. Contraindications include chronic alcoholism, drug and substance abuse, major psychiatric disorder, severe gastroesophageal reflux disease and chronic duodenal ulcer.

2.2. Preoperative work up and preparation

Comprehensive preoperative workup for sleeve gastrectomy is the same as that of the other bariatric procedures. Patients are admitted the day prior to the procedure when they are started on clear liquid diet. Single dose of prophylactic antibiotic and proton pump inhibitor are given an hour prior to surgery. Low molecular-weight heparin (LMWH) is prescribed to lower the incidence of deep vein thrombosis (DVT) and other thromboembolic events, till the patient is ambulated.

2.3. Operative technique

2.3.1. Positioning

Patient is positioned flat on the operating table with both upper extremities extended out. Patient is secured at the chest and thighs using straps and a foot board in preparation for a steep reverse Trendelenburg position. The surgeon and the scrub nurse both stand on the patient's right while the first assistant and the cameraman stand on the patient's left.

2.3.2. Port placement

A three-four ports technique is utilized for this procedure as shown in **Figure 1**. Pneumoperitoneum is created by Veress needle or optical trocar is used at the first port. The first port is about three finger breadths to the left of umbilicus, at about 20 cm from the xiphisternum. The second 15 mm port is inserted at supraumbilical site. Another 5 mm trocar is inserted in the right midclavicular line below the costal margin, for surgeon's left hand, such that the falciform ligament does not cause difficulty in dissection of the hiatus. Lastly an optional 5 mm assistant port can be placed in the left anterior axillary line just below the costal margin.

2.3.3. Placement of liver suspension tape

To elevate the central and left lobe of the liver, a liver suspension tape (LST) was designed. Two pieces of Jackson-Pratt (JP) drain measuring 2 cm each were cut and fixed with 2/0 polypropylene suture (Ethicon W8400 2-0 Prolene blue 70 mm round bodied). The lateral segment of the left lobe was suspended using the tape by passing the needle through the liver, out through the anterior abdominal wall and secured with clamps. Another LST was inserted in the medial aspect of left lobe of liver to retract the liver completely.

The LSTs should not be placed more than 2 cm away from the liver edge to achieve optimal retraction and prevent major bile duct or vessel injury (**Figure 2**). Alternatively, a Nathanson

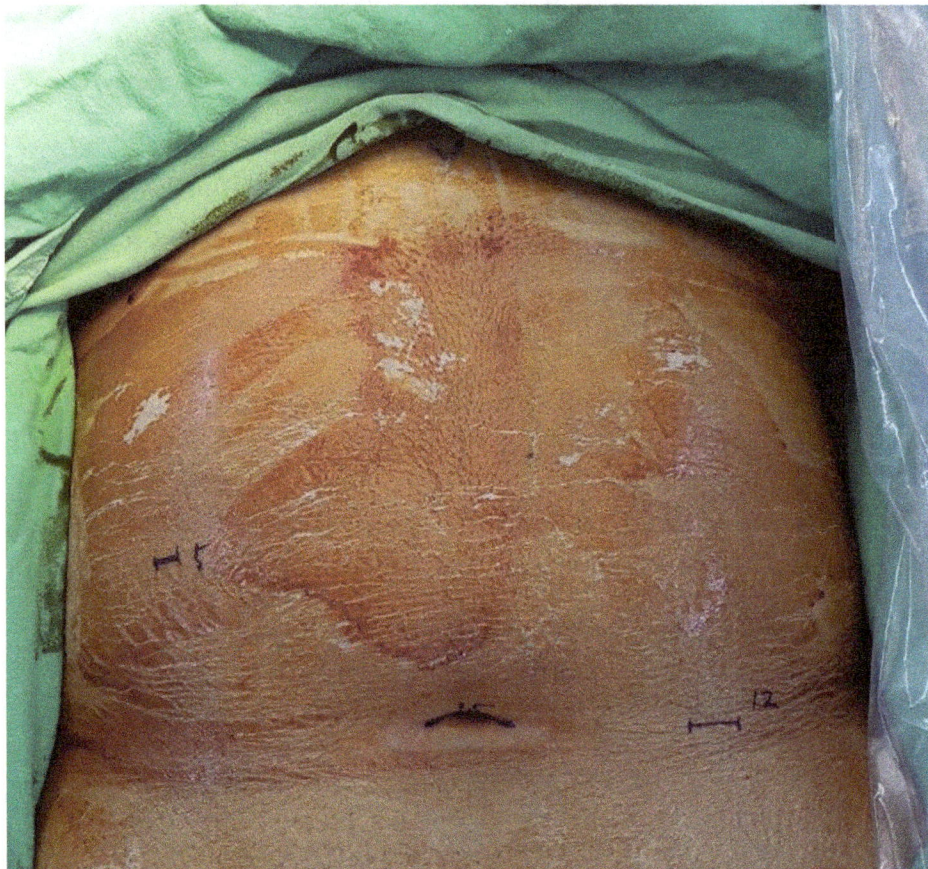

Figure 1. Port placement for LSG.

liver retractor (C-NLRS-1001 Cook Medical) may be used in order to achieve good exposure of the entire length of the stomach and duodenum. This may be placed using a 5 mm port inserted in the subxiphoid area.

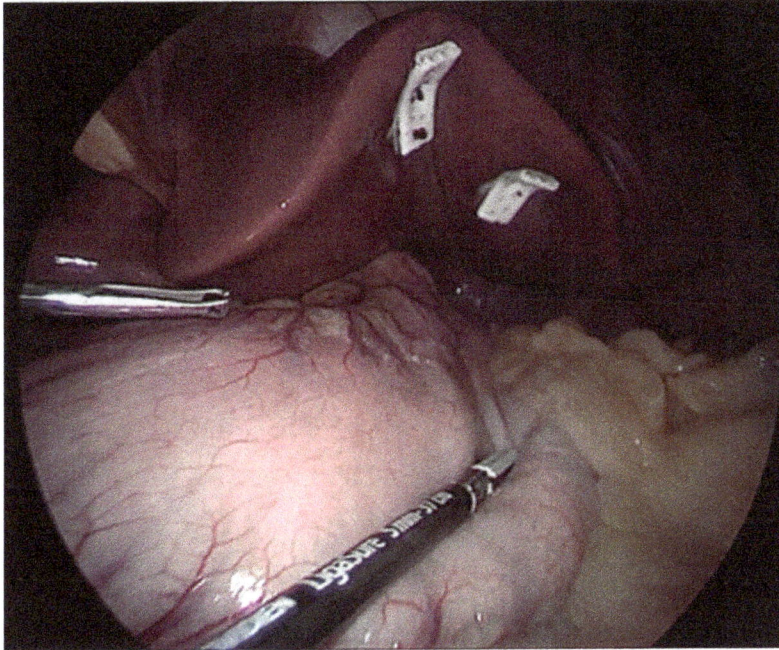

Figure 2. Retraction of left lobe of liver with liver suspension tape.

2.3.4. Mobilization of the gastrocolic ligament

Dissection of the gastrocolic ligament close to the greater curvature of the stomach commences at a point opposite the incisura angularis. A window in the lesser sac is created and dissection is started using a vessel sealing energy device (Ligasure™ vessel sealing device by Covidien-Medtronic or Harmonic Ace by Ethicon). By staying very close to the gastric wall, the entire gastrocolic ligament is detached up to the angle of His taking care at the area of the short gastric vessels at the splenic hilum (**Figures 3** and **4**). Care should be taken not to injure left gastric vessels.

2.3.5. Dissection at the angle of His

Fundus of the stomach must be mobilized from its adhesions and completely resected. A very useful anatomical landmark is to expose the left crus of the hiatus. Dissection of the left crus is terminated once the left phrenoesophageal ligament has been completely visualized (**Figure 5**). The posterior attachments of the fundus to the anterior border of the pancreas are completely mobilized to properly identify and preserve the left gastric vessels (**Figure 6**).

The anterior portion of the gastroesophageal fat pad (Belsey's pad of fat) is then dissected in order to expose half of the anterior portion of the GE junction. Care is taken not to completely devascularize this fat pad which may increase the rate of leak at the GE junction.

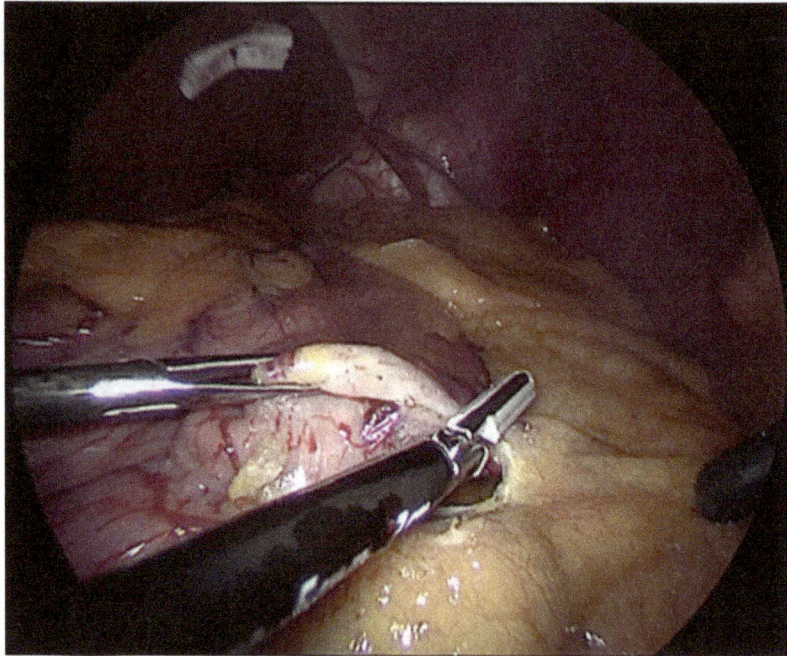

Figure 3. Start of dissection by creating a window in the lesser sac.

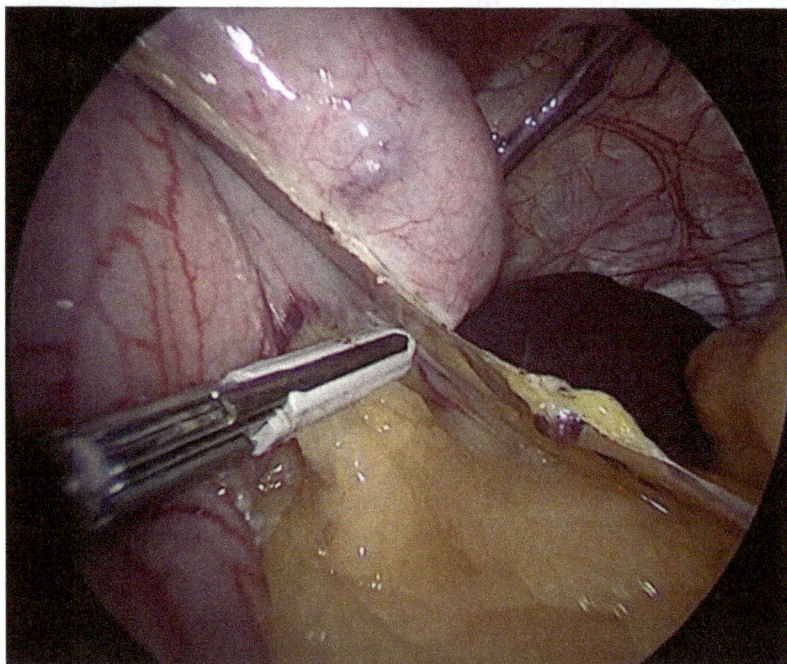

Figure 4. Dissection of the gastrocolic ligament at short gastric vessels near splenic hilum.

2.3.6. Dissection of the caudal part of the gastrocolic ligament

The gastrocolic ligament at the area of the right gastroepiploic vessel is dissected caudally till the distance of 4 cm from the pylorus. Dense adhesions around the prepyloric area may be encountered and should be taken down individually (**Figure 7**).

2.3.7. Sleeve gastrectomy

Prior to the creation of the actual sleeve, make sure that the entire stomach is laid down flat. At this point, the anesthesiologist inserts an orogastric tube with its tip positioned by the surgeon under direct visual guidance. Using an L-hook dissector (STORZ 37370DL Monopolar Dissecting L-Hook Cannula), marking on the anterior surface of the stomach is done which

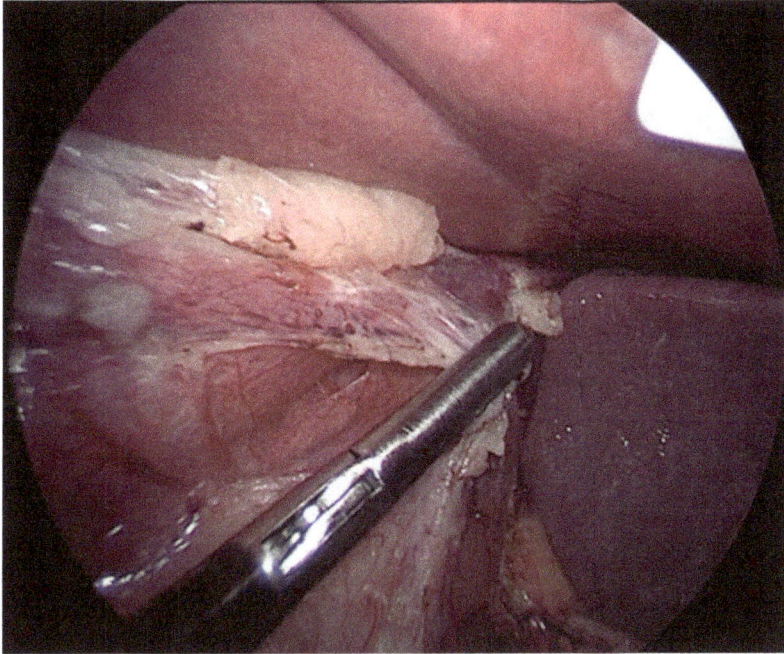

Figure 5. Dissection at the angle of His exposing the left crus and phrenoesophageal ligament.

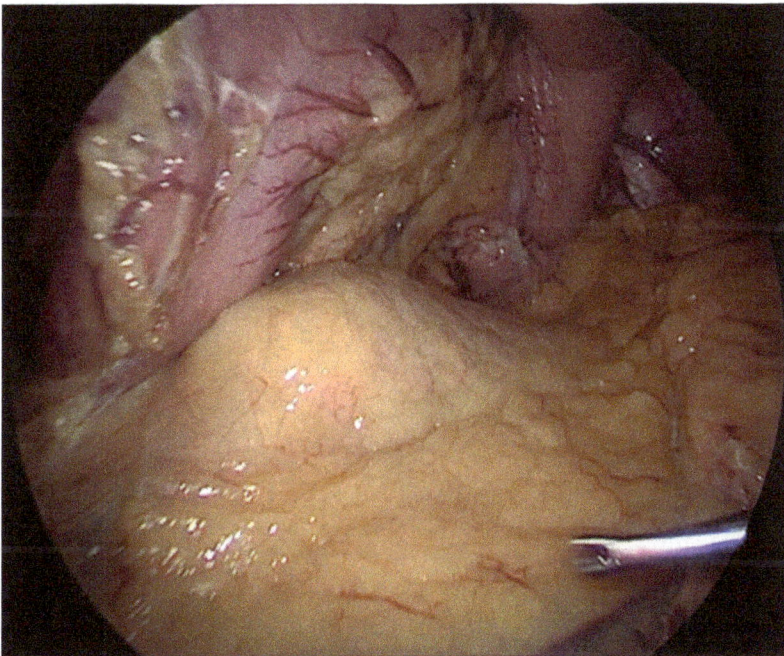

Figure 6. Complete mobilization of the posterior attachments of the fundus and anterior border of the pancreas.

will serve as a guide for the surgeon to place the endostapler with 38 Fr orogastric tube as stent (**Figure 8**). For the first staple firing, the stapling device is placed 4 cm away from the pylorus and 2.5–3 cm away from the incisura angularis in order to prevent narrowing (**Figure 9**). A black 60 mm reload (EGIA60AXT Endo GIA 60 mm articulating extra-thick reload with Tri-Staple Technology) or a green 60 mm green reload (ECR60G Echelon Endopath stapler reload cartridges by Ethicon) using manual or powered device is used. Successive firings

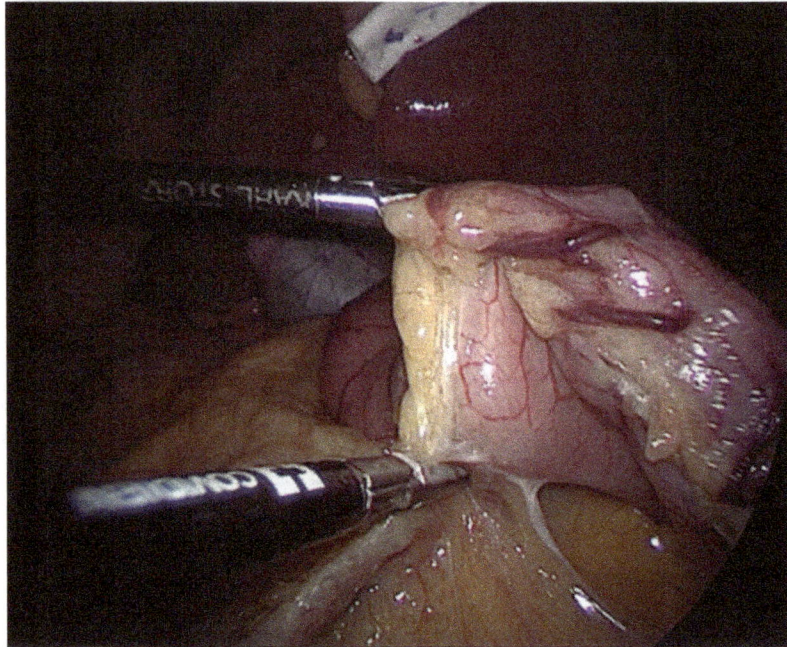

Figure 7. Dissection of the gastrocolic ligament toward the pylorus.

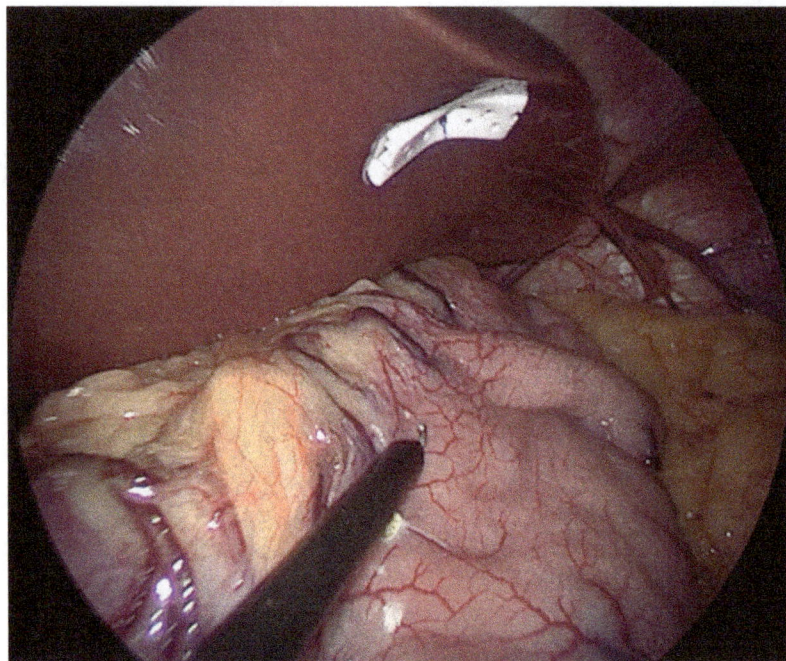

Figure 8. Marking of the transection line along the anterior surface of the stomach.

of the stapling device toward the gastric fundus are done using either a 60 mm purple cartridge (EGIA60AMT Endo GIA 60 mm articulating medium/thick reload with Tri-Staple Technology) or a 60 mm blue cartridge (ETHECR60B Echelon Endopath stapler reload cartridges by Ethicon) (**Figure 10**). Commencing after placement of the second stapler, loose migratory crotch staples must be removed in order to prevent improper formation of the

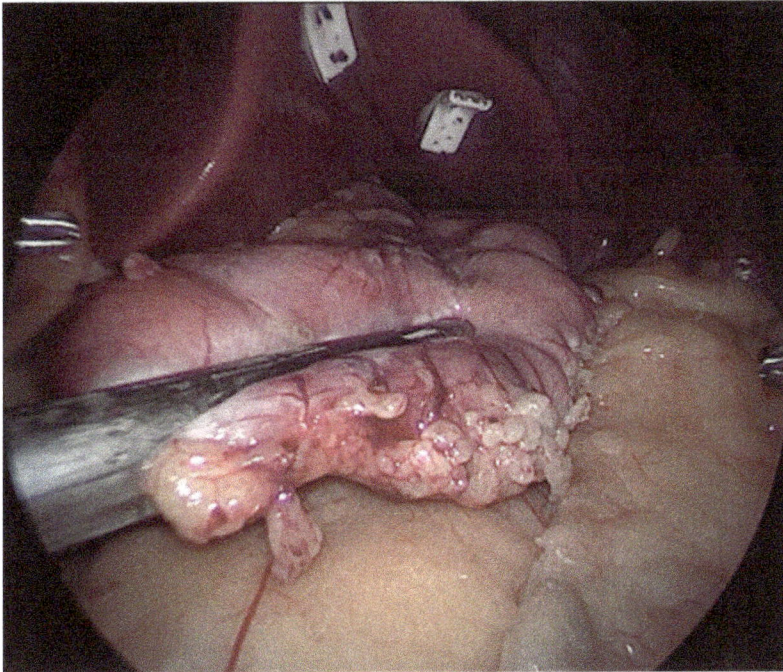

Figure 9. First staple firing 4 cm from pylorus and 2.5–3 cm away from the incisura.

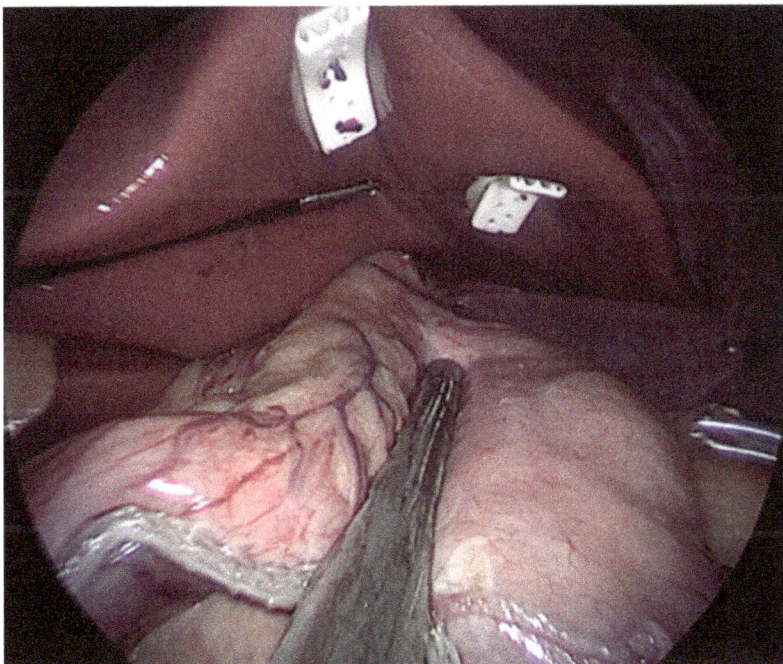

Figure 10. Successive firings of the staple device toward the fundus.

suture line (**Figure 11**). Constant communication with the anesthesiologist is of paramount importance, inserting and withdrawing the orogastric tube before and after application of each stapler to make sure the bougie is not stapled into the remnant stomach. It is also highly recommended to check the posterior aspect of the stomach before each firing of the device in order to avoid twisting and in-folding of tissues. The entire fundus, including its posterior

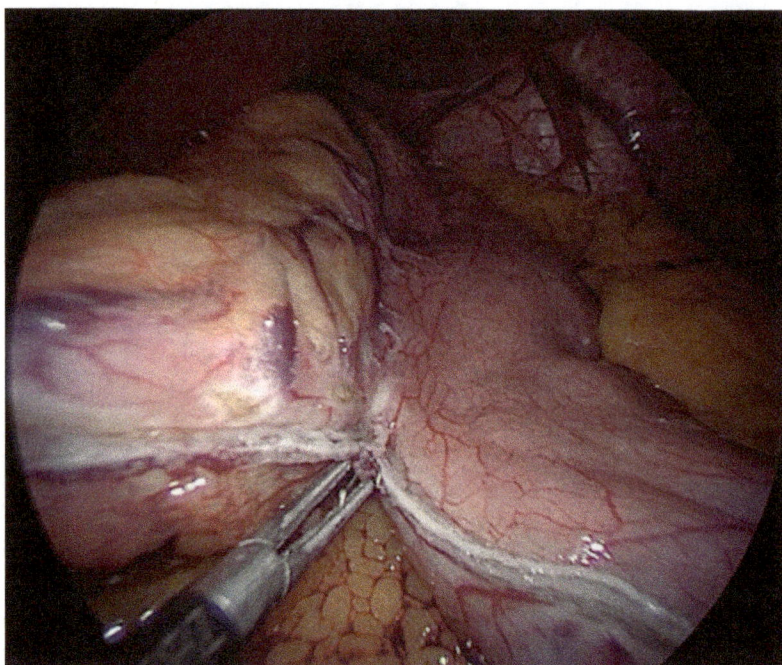

Figure 11. Removal of migratory crotch staples.

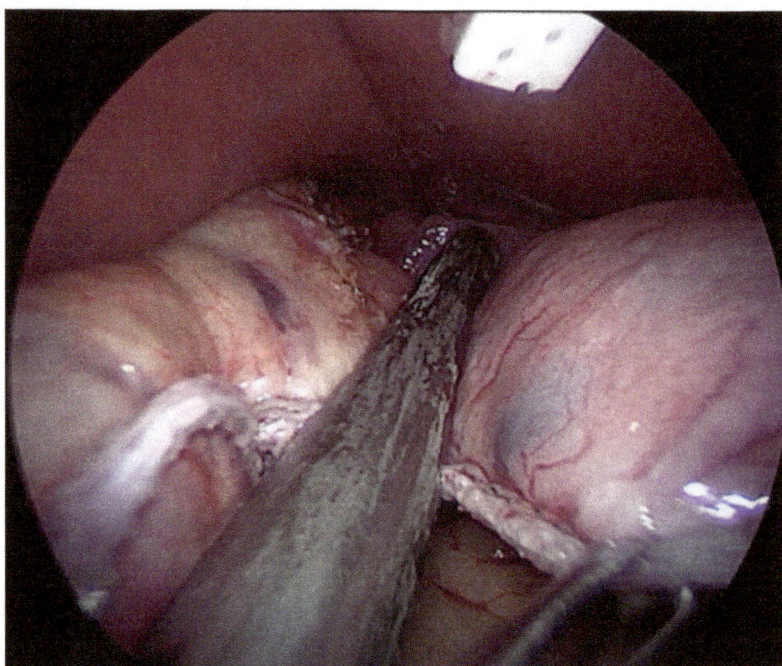

Figure 12. Staple firing 1 cm away from the GE junction.

wall, is to be included in the resected part. Before firing of the last stapler, always verify that the stapler is placed not less than 1 cm from the GE junction and that both tips of the stapler are always in sight (**Figure 12**).

2.3.8. Hemostasis

The entire length of the staple line should be inspected for any bleeding. Bleeding may be controlled using electrocautery, clips or over sewing. No buttressing material is placed over the staple line.

2.3.9. Fixing the tube

One or two fixing stitches are taken between the stapled sleeve and the retroperitoneal fat to prevent rotation of the sleeve tube.

2.3.10. Specimen extraction

The LSTs are removed and the entry and exit points on the liver are cauterized to achieve hemostasis. Specimen is then extracted through the umbilical port and closure of the rectus sheath done with 2-0 Vicryl. Subcutaneous layers of all ports closed with 3-0 Vicryl and skin closed with interrupted subcuticular stitches. Dermabond is applied and dressing done.

2.3.11. Surgical outcomes

The mechanism of action of LSG appears to be by the restriction of the volume of stomach and the removal of ghrelin-producing fundus [3]. The decreased ghrelin leads to early satiety and decreased hunger. Another mechanism is increased gastric emptying which combined with decreased gastric acid secretion causes incomplete digestion [4]. Increased gastric emptying is associated with higher levels of glucagon-like-peptide-1 (GLP-1), a glucose-regulating insulin-enhancing agent, which has been linked to weight loss and resolution of type 2 diabetes mellitus [5].

In a retrospective study, the EWL after 3 and 6 years follow-up of LSG was 72.8 and 57.3%, respectively [4]. Gustavo et al. in their long-term study showed a mean %EBMIL (percentage of excess BMI Loss) of 82.4, 75.9 and 62.5 and % TWL (percentage of total weight loss) of 28.5, 25.8 and 21 at 3, 6 and 11+ years of follow-up, respectively [6].

3. Sleeve-based procedures

One of the arguments against LSG is that its weight loss as well as its efficacy in diabetes remission is inferior and not sustainable compared to RYGB. This is owed to the fact that LSG do not own the content of bowel bypass. Laparoscopic loop duodenojejunal bypass with sleeve gastrectomy (LDJB-SG) and sleeve gastrectomy with proximal jejunal bypass (SG-PJB) are a combination of both a restrictive and malabsorptive procedures (**Figure 13** and **28**). First described by Huang et al. in 2011, LDJB-SG has a lower incidence of dumping syndrome and marginal ulcer, both commonly experienced in RYGB, due to an intact pylorus which acts as

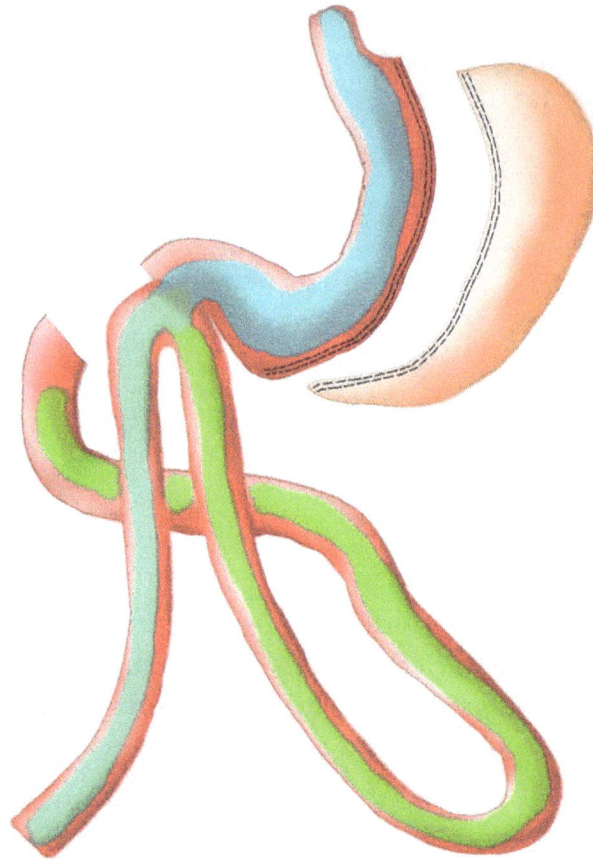

Figure 13. Schematic diagram of LDJB-SG.

a sphincter mechanism and a creates a neutral condition from mixture of gastric acid, pancreatic juice and bile around the duodenojejunal anastomosis [7]. SG-PJB was designed by Alamo et al. in 2005 and later revised in 2009 [9, 10]. Surgical results of weight loss and comorbidity resolution were comparable to Roux-en-Y gastric bypass in his reports. Both LDJB-SG and SGPJB can be an alternative operation that could potentially lessen the complications associated with the conventional gastric bypass.

3.1. Loop DuodenoJejunal Bypass with Sleeve Gastrectomy

3.1.1. Indications and Contraindications

Indication for this procedure includes BMI ≥ 40 kg/m^2 without comorbidities or ≥ 35 kg/m^2. This can also be offered as a surgical treatment for poorly controlled type 2 diabetes in Asian patients with BMI ≥ 32.5 kg/m^2 without comorbidities or >27.5 kg/m^2 with comorbidities. Contraindications include chronic alcoholism, drug and substance abuse, major psychiatric disorder, severe gastroesophageal reflux disease and chronic duodenal ulcer [8].

3.1.2. Preoperative work up and preparation

Comprehensive preoperative workup for DJB-SG is the same as that of the other bariatric procedures. Patients are admitted the day prior to the procedure were they are started on clear liquid diet. Single dose of prophylactic antibiotic and proton pump inhibitor are given an hour prior to surgery. Low molecular-weight heparin (LMWH) is prescribed to lower the incidence of deep vein thrombosis (DVT) and other thromboembolic events.

3.1.3. Positioning

Patient is positioned flat on the operating table with both upper extremities extended out. Patient is secured at the chest and thighs using straps and a foot board in preparation for a steep reverse Trendelenburg position. The surgeon and the scrub nurse both stand on the patient's right while the first assistant and the cameraman stand on the patient's left.

3.1.4. Operative Technique

3.1.4.1. Port placement

Five-port technique is utilized for this procedure as shown in **Figure 14**. A 12 mm optical port on the left of umbilicus is placed after abdominal cavity is entered using the closed Veress technique or via an optical trocar. One 15 mm port is placed in immediate supraumbilical region and another 12 mm port is placed to the right of umbilicus mirroring the one on the left, both of which serve as the surgeon's right hand working ports. A 5 mm trocar is placed in the right midclavicular line below the costal margin for the surgeon's left hand while another 5 mm trocar is placed in the midclavicular line below the left subcostal margin for the assistant.

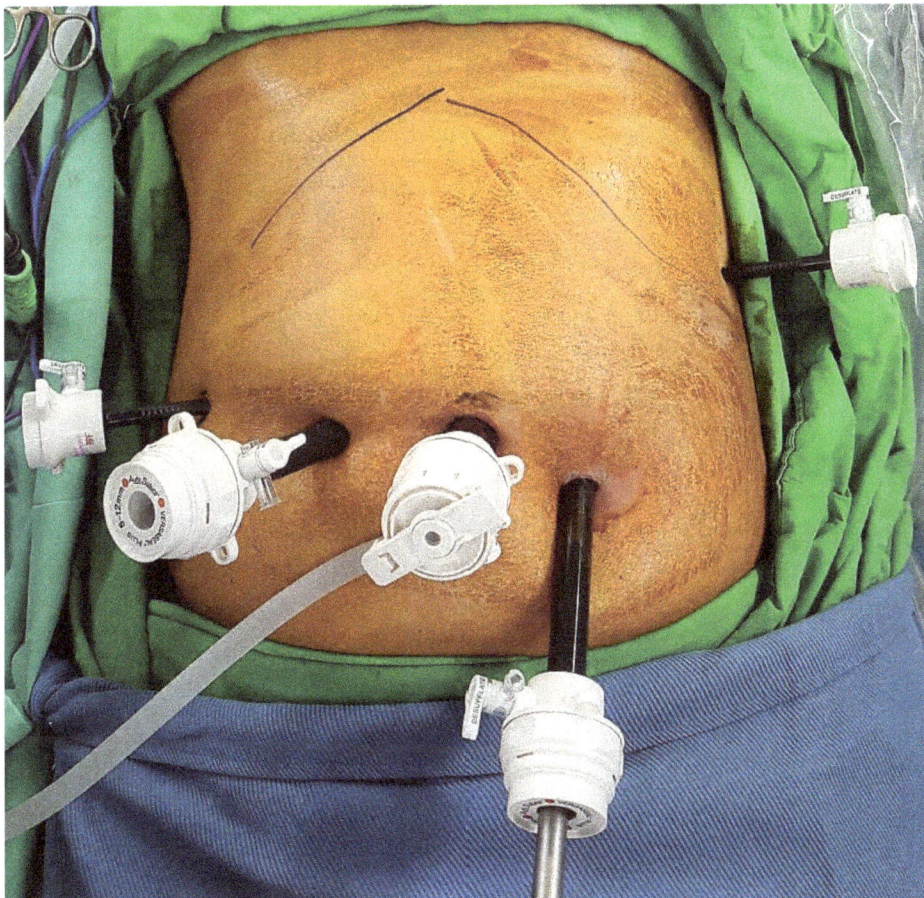

Figure 14. Port placement for LDJB-SG.

3.1.4.2. Placement of liver suspension tape

An LST previously discussed earlier in this chapter is utilized. However, instead of using a 2.5 cm cut JP drain, 5 cm is used for the second tape in order to lift both the lobes of the liver along with the falciform ligament away from the field (**Figure 15**).

3.1.4.3. Sleeve gastrectomy

The formation of the gastric sleeve tube is done in a similar way as described earlier in this chapter.

3.1.4.4. Duodenal transection

Proper exposure of the entire length of the stomach and first part of the duodenum is critical to the success of this procedure. After sleeve gastrectomy has been performed, the next step is to dissect the first part of the duodenum. A counter traction suture is placed at the distal end of the sleeved stomach to visualize the first part of the duodenum (**Figure 16**). At a distance approximately 2 cm distal to the pylorus, a tunnel is created posterior to the duodenal wall and just anterior to the gastroduodenal artery using a combination of a blunt dissector and Flexlap Gold Finger retractor (Flexlap Gold Finger Retractor by Ethicon Endo Surgery, USA) as seen in **Figures 17** and **18**. A tape is then passed in the tunnel behind the duodenum and lifted laterally and downwards to serve as a traction while inserting the endostapler (**Figure 19**). Using a 45 mm curved tip articulating tan reload (EGIA45CTAVM Endo GIA 45 mm Curved Tip articulating vascular/medium reload with Tri-Staple™ Technology), the first part of the duodenum is transected. Care is taken to avoid injury to the common bile duct (CBD), pancreas and major vessels in the area (**Figure 20**) [8].

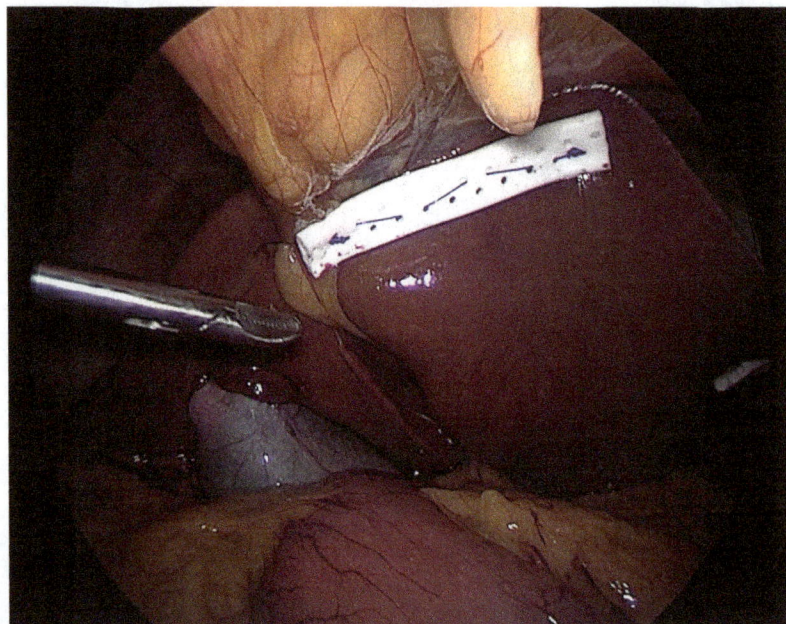

Figure 15. Liver suspension for both lobes.

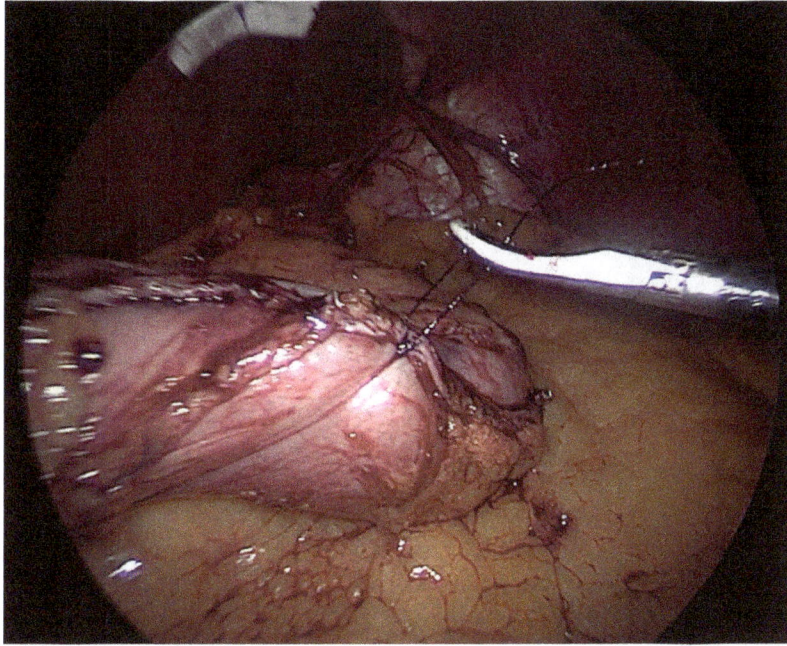

Figure 16. Counter traction suture.

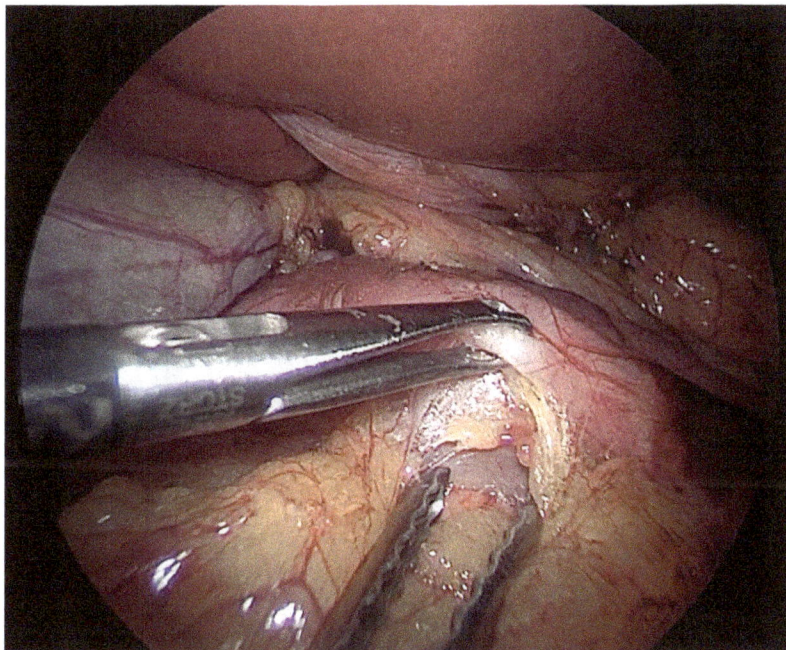

Figure 17. Retroduodenal tunnel.

3.1.4.5. Duodenojejunostomy

The ligament of Treitz is identified as it exits at the root of the transverse mesocolon. A length of jejunum is measured for 200–300 cm starting from the ligament of Treitz. The loop of jejunum is pulled up and a stay suture is placed between the loop of jejunum and pylorus. An enterotomy of 1.5 cm is placed obliquely in the first part of the duodenum and antimesenteric

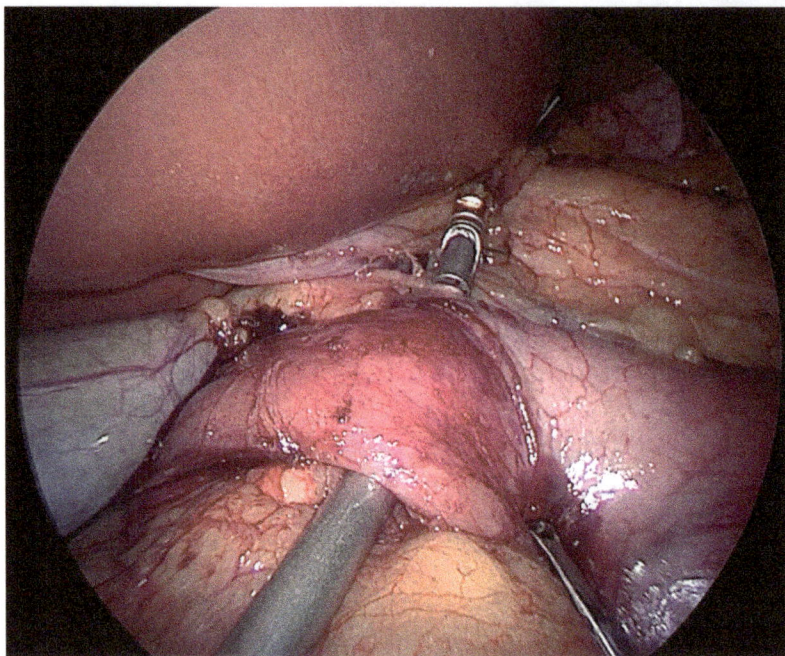

Figure 18. Retroduodenal tunnel passing through the lesser sac using the Goldfinger retractor.

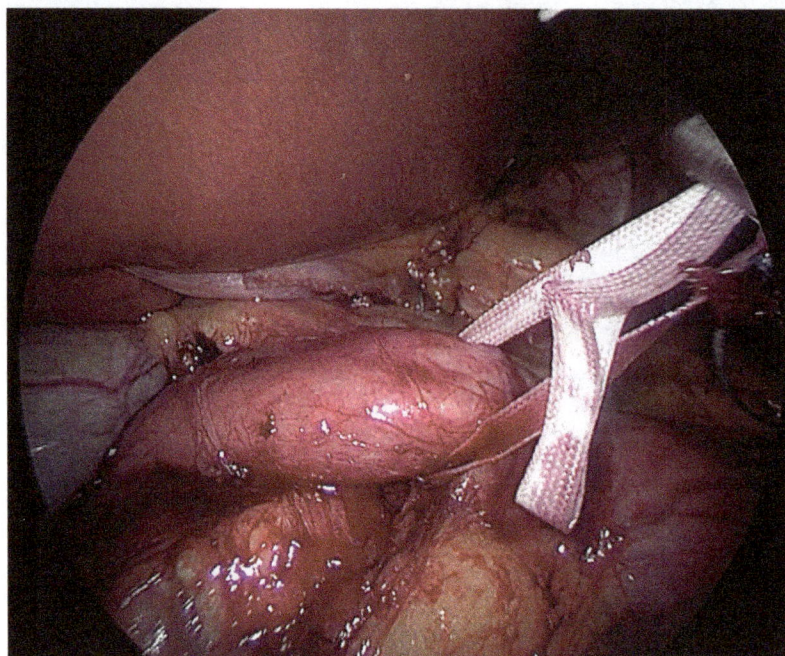

Figure 19. Lifting and retraction of the 1st portion of the duodenum using a tape.

side of jejunum (**Figure 21** and **22**). A completely hand-sewn side to side duodenojejunal anastomosis in a running fashion is created using a 3-0 absorbable glyconate monofilament suture (3-0 B I BRAUN MONOSYN™ UNDYED 28" HR26 TAPER) (**Figures 23–25**). Then an antitorsion suture between antrum and jejunum is placed, around 4 cm proximal to the D-J anastomosis [8].

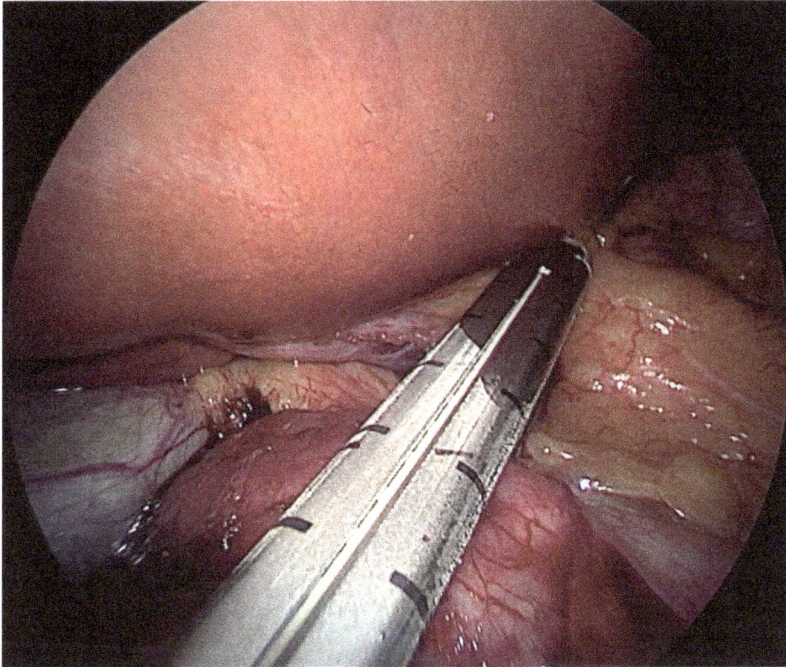

Figure 20. Duodenal transection.

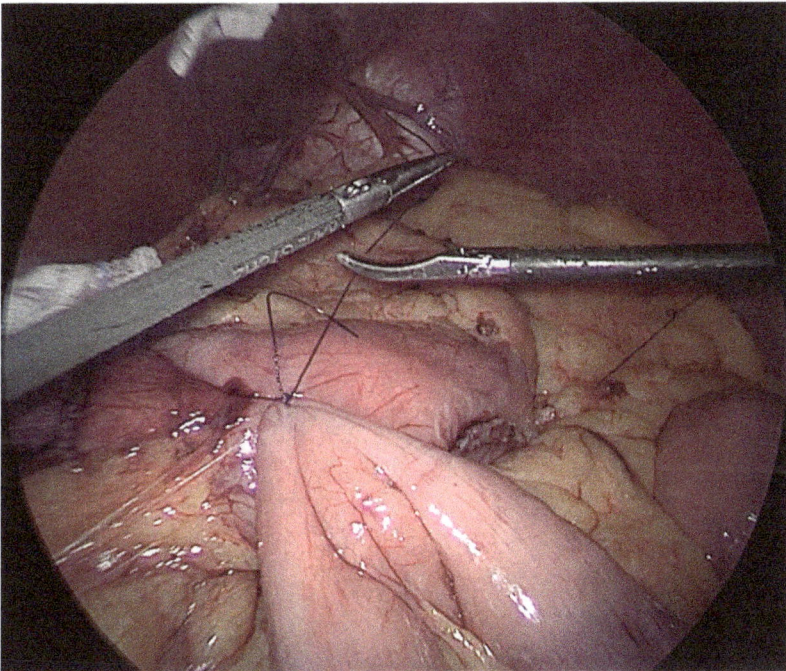

Figure 21. Stay suture between sleeved stomach and jejunum.

3.1.4.6. Closure of mesenteric defect

Peterson's mesenteric defect is closed in a continuous running technique using 2-0 nonabsorbable polyester suture (W6977 Ethibond Excel™ Polyester suture) (**Figure 26**). A Jackson Pratt drain is placed under the entire length of stomach tube and duodenojejunal anastomosis (**Figure 27**).

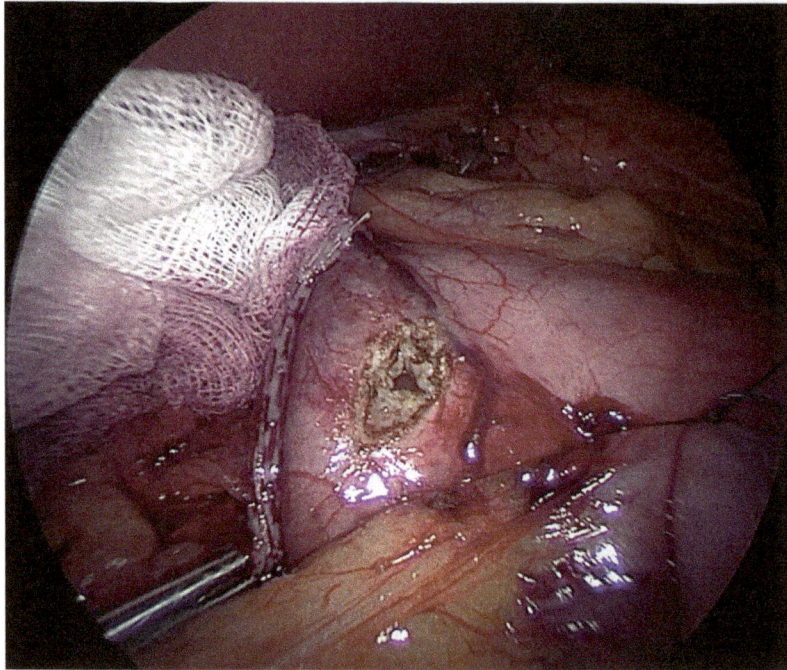

Figure 22. Duodenal enterotomy placed obliquely.

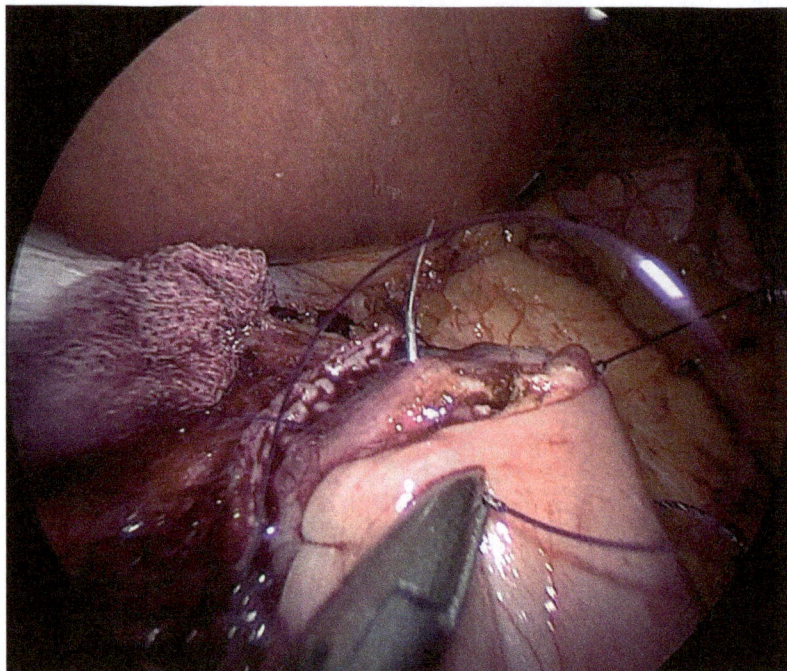

Figure 23. Completely hand-sewn duodenojejunal bypass.

3.1.4.7. Postoperative care and follow-up

Adhering to the early recovery after surgery (ERAS) postoperative protocol, adequate pain control is administered via the intravenous route and early ambulation is encouraged in our patients as early as six hours after surgery in order to avoid pulmonary complications.

Once the patient is fully awake, clear liquid diet as instructed by our dietitian is commenced. Intravenous antibiotic is administered for one more day. Patients are usually discharged 2–3 days after surgery. Patients are placed on bariatric diet as instructed by the dietitian. Proton pump inhibitors are given for 1 month after surgery. Follow-up schedule is as follows: 1 week, 1, 3, 6 and 12 months after surgery. One year after the surgery, patients are advised to follow-up every 6 months thereafter.

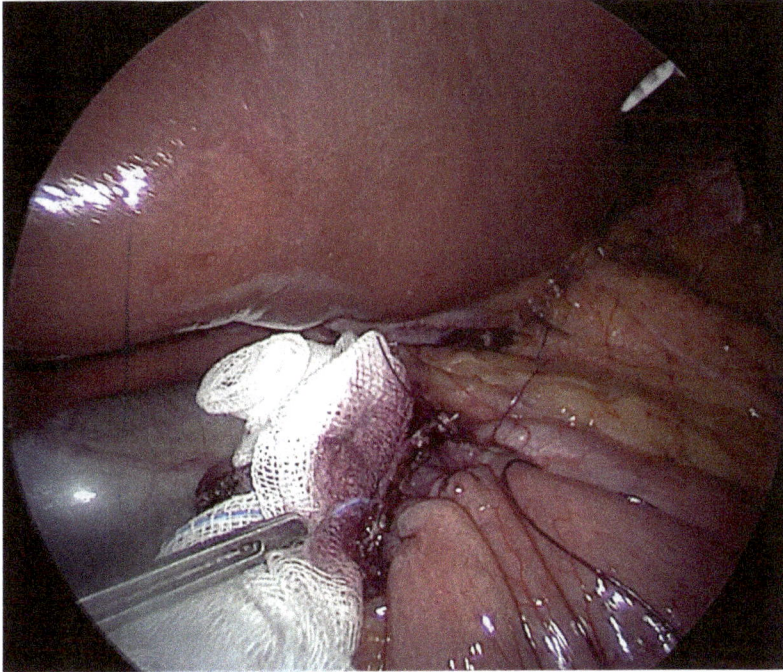

Figure 24. Anterior wall of DJB.

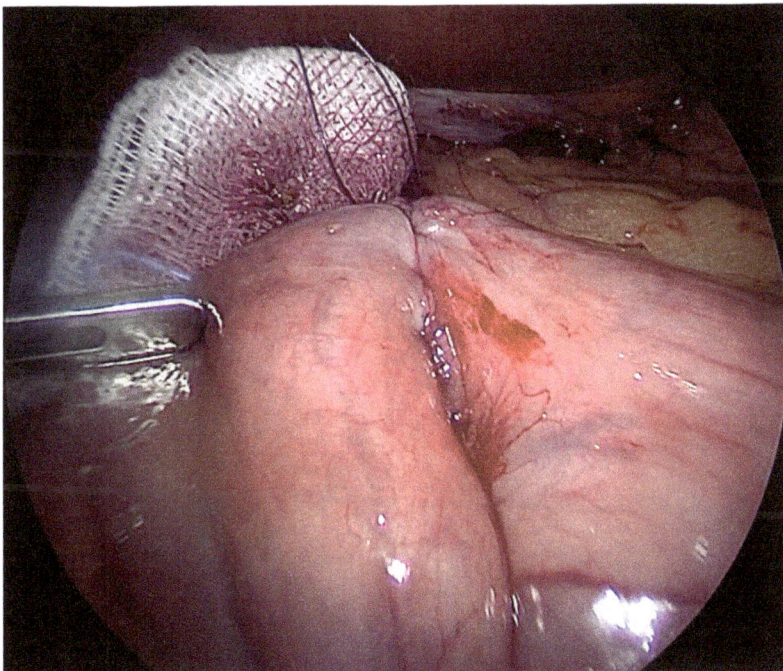

Figure 25. Posterior wall of DJB.

3.1.5. Surgical Outcomes

The mechanism of weight loss in LDJB-SG is due to the resection of Ghrelin-secreting cells located in the fundus of the stomach. A significant drop in this hormone's level after the procedure causes decrease in sensation of hunger and early satiety. Furthermore, aside from its weight-loss effect, caloric restriction also helps in the improvement of insulin resistance and

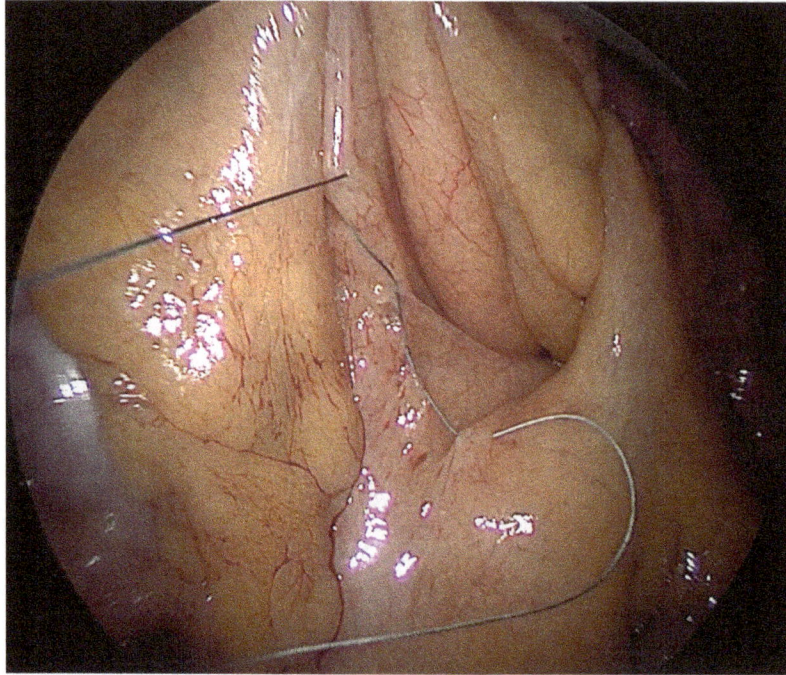

Figure 26. Closure of Petersons defect.

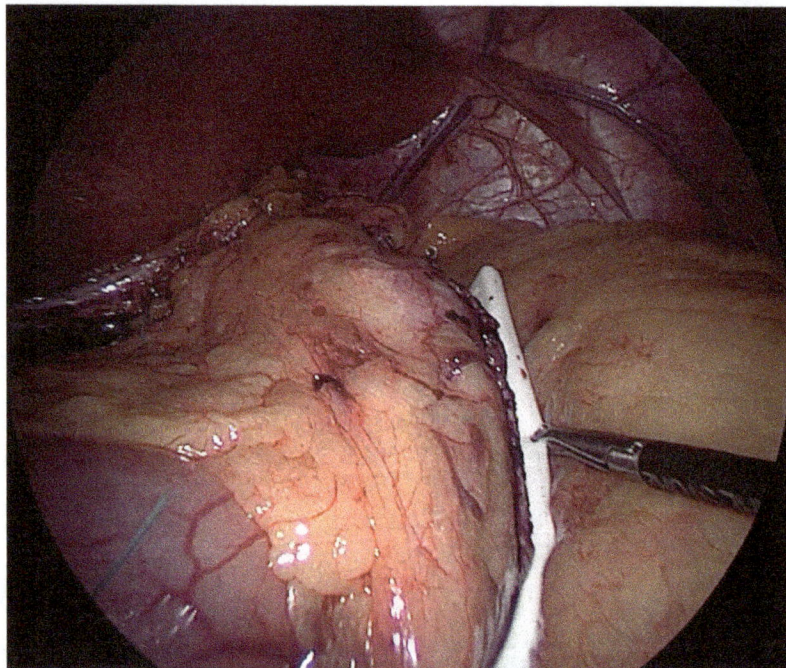

Figure 27. Placement of JP drain along DJB anastomosis and entire length of the sleeve suture line.

increase in glucose tolerance. However, the efficient glycemic control of this procedure is predominantly due to the exclusion of the duodenum (Foregut theory) and the faster delivery of undigested food and more concentrated bile to the distal small bowel (Hindgut theory) which ensures secretion of incretins.

In a prospective study by Huang et al. published in 2013 comparing LDJB-SG with RYGB, LDJB-SG had a superior remission rate of T2DM (60% vs 49%) and a better over-all glycemic control (90% vs 71%) compared to RYGB in patients with BMI $\leq$ 35 kg/m^2 at 1 year after surgery. Fasting blood sugar levels was also significantly lower in the LDJB-SG group (98.0 ± 18.0 vs 106.0 ± 31.7 mg/dl). The drop in HbA1C was also lower in the LDJB-SG compared to the RYGB (6.0 ± 0.9 vs 6.3 ± 1.2) although this did not attain a statistically significant level (P value = 0.442). Resolution of other obesity-related comorbid factors were also seen in LDJB-SG that was comparable to the RYGB group (Hypertension = 85.7% vs 88.2% and Dyslipidemia = 70% vs 76.6% resolution rates) [8].

In a case-matched study comparing of 30 patients undergoing LDJB-SG and 30 patients undergoing RYGB, the mean BMIs dropped significantly to 22.4 kg/m^2 (±2.4) (range 18.4–27 kg/m^2) and 21.9 kg/m^2 (±2.5) (range 17.7–26.5 kg/m^2) from preoperative values of 28.2 kg/m^2 (±3.6) and 27.8 kg/m^2 (±3.8) at 1 year after surgery (p < 0.01). However, no statistical difference was seen between the two groups. HbA1c and fasting glucose were also significantly decreased 1 year after surgery compared to its preoperative value from 8.98 (±1.75%) to 6.52% (±1.03) and 168.3 (±54.9 mg/dL) to 106.5 mg/dL (±28.2 mg/dL). Comparing complete remission of T2DM in 1 year after surgery, the LDJB-SG had a remission rate of 36.6% of patients (11/30) compared to 30% (9/30) in the RYGB group. As far as complications, the rate for early complication favors that of RYGB (1 case vs 4 cases). However, there is a note of a trend toward lower occurrence of late complication rate in LDJB-SG compared to RYGB (5 vs 8 cases, p < 0.08) [11].

Lee et al. compared single anastomosis duodenojejunal bypass with sleeve gastrectomy (SADJB-SG) with RYGB and minigastric bypass (MGB). The operation time was significantly longer in SADJB-SG compared to the other types of bypass (181.7 mins vs 160 mins for RYGB vs 120.1 mins for MGB; p < 0.01). During the interim follow up period at 1, 3, 6 and 12 months after surgery, the mean BMI dropped to 32.9 ± 4.8, 29.9 ± 6.8, 27.6 ± 5.4 and 25.9 ± 4.6 kg/m^2, respectively. The percentage weight loss during these same follow-up periods were 15.1, 20.3 25 and 32.7%. 12 months after surgery, comparing percent weight loss (% WL) of the three procedures, the results showed a higher percent weight loss for SADJB-SG (32.7 ± 7.9% SADJB-SG vs 28.9 ± 9.0% MGB vs 26.1 ± 4.1% RYGB). Results also showed a superior percent excess weight loss for SADJB-SG (80.3 ± 24.8%) compared to the two bypass procedures (68.6 ± 58.2% MGB and 63.4 ± 31.8% RYGB). In the same report, T2DM was seen in > 80% of the subjects with a preoperative mean HbA1c level of 9.2%. This value decreased to 6.1% 1 year after surgery with a complete remission rate of T2DM in 64% of the patients [12].

In an attempt to evaluate the role of duodenal exclusion in glycemic control, a matched group study comparing LDJB-SG and SG alone was done. At 1 year after surgery, the LDJB-SG (26 patients) presented with a higher percent excess weight loss (87.2 ± 14.9% vs 67 ± 27.0%; p = 0.23) and a lower BMI (23.9 ± 2.2 vs 26.1 ± 3.7; p = 0.065) compared to the SG alone group (29 patients). As far as T2DM remission rate is concerned, the LDJB-SG had a 92.3% total glycemic control rate compared to 86.2% in the SG alone group. The mean reduction in the HbA1c level for the LDJB-SG was likewise higher compared to the SG group (2.8 vs 2.1% p = 0.45) [13].

3.2. Sleeve gastrectomy with proximal jejunal bypass (Figure 28)

3.2.1. Indication and contraindication

The indications and contraindications of PJB-SG are the same as that of the conventional stand-alone sleeve gastrectomy. Furthermore, this can also be offered as a metabolic surgery for patients with BMI between 27.5 and 35 with type 2 Diabets.

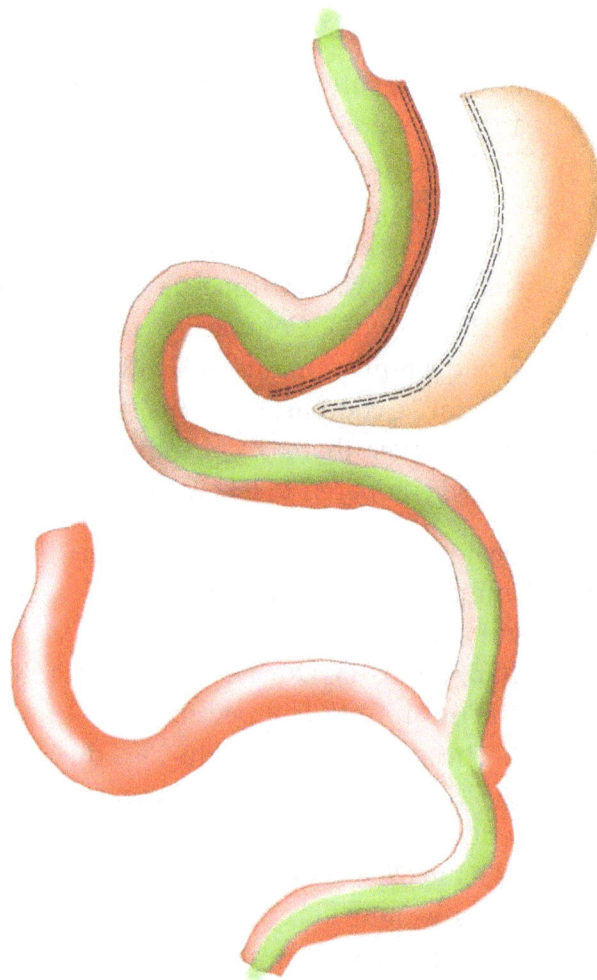

Figure 28. Schematic diagram of LPJB-SG.

3.2.2. Preoperative workup and preparation

Like in all bariatric procedures, a complete preoperative workup should be done in order to select appropriate candidates for the procedure. All patients are evaluated by a multidisciplinary team dedicated in bariatric surgery including a bariatric surgeon, bariatric physician, gastroen-terologist, anesthesiologist, psychiatrist, nutritionist and fitness coach. Other specialists may be called upon if required.

3.2.3. Positioning

Patient is positioned supine with upper extremities abducted and lower extremities adducted. Patient is then secured to the operating table using straps and foot boards. Patient is placed in steep reverse Trendelenburg position.

3.2.4. Operative technique

3.2.4.1. Port placement

A 4-port technique is utilized with the surgeon positioned on the patient's right side and the assistant and camera man standing on the patient's left. Port placement is similar to LSG with an assistant port in left anterior axillary line below the costal margin **(Figure 29)**.

3.2.4.2. Pneumoperitoneum

Pneumoperitoneum is accomplished either via Veress technique or through a 12 mm optical trocar using a 30-degree scope in the left periumbilical area.

3.2.4.3. Placement of liver suspension tape

Liver retraction is done using the LST similarly placed as in the standard LSG technique. Alternatively, a Nathanson liver retractor can also be used.

3.2.4.4. Sleeve gastrectomy

Standard sleeve gastrectomy is performed as previously described earlier in this chapter.

3.2.4.5. Proximal jejunal bypass

After completing the sleeve gastrectomy, ligament of Treitz is identified. Transection of the jejunum is done at 20 cm from the ligament of Treitz using either a 45 mm white cartridge reload (EGIA45AMT Endo GIA™ 45 mm articulating medium/thick reload with Tri-Staple Technology) or a 45 mm white cartridge reload (ECR45W Echelon Endopath™ tri-stapler reload cartridges by Ethicon). Next 300 cm of small bowel is measured distally and a side-to-side jejunojejunal anastomosis was fashioned out using the same cartridge and stapling device. The jejunojejunostomy is created with hand-sewn technique using 3-0 Absorbable Glyconate Monofilament running suture (3-0 B I BRAUN MONOSYN™ UNDYED 28" HR26 TAPER) **(Figures 30–32)**.

3.2.4.6. Closure of mesenteric defect

The mesenteric defect is closed with simple running sutures using 2-0 nonabsorbable polyes-ter suture (Ethibond Excel™ polyester suture). No drain is placed.

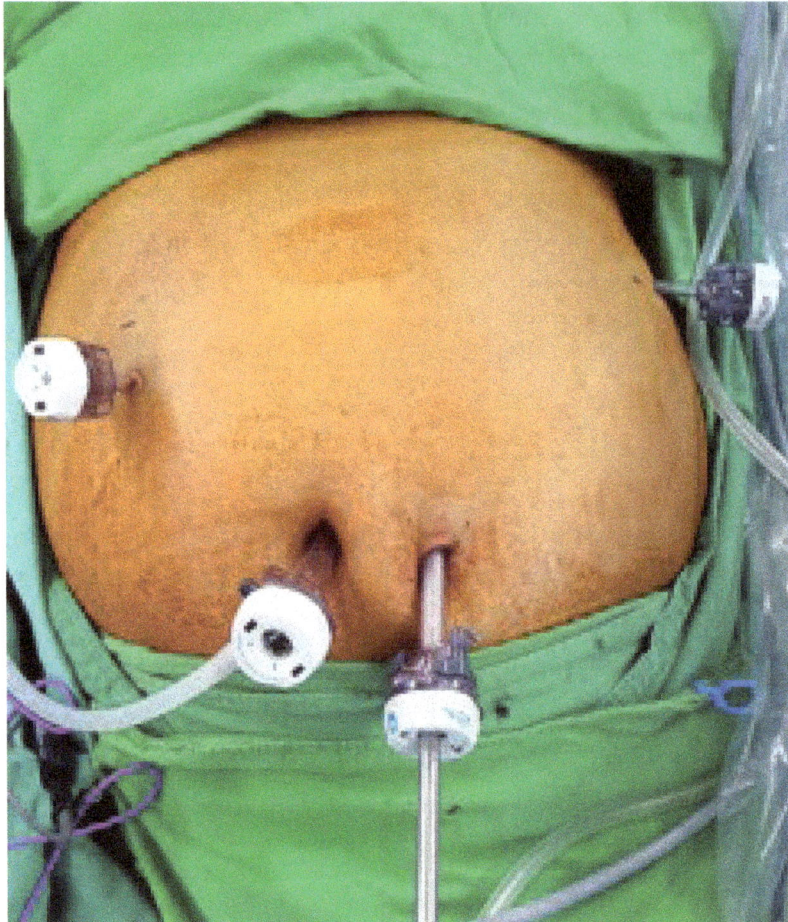

Figure 29. LPJB-SG port placement.

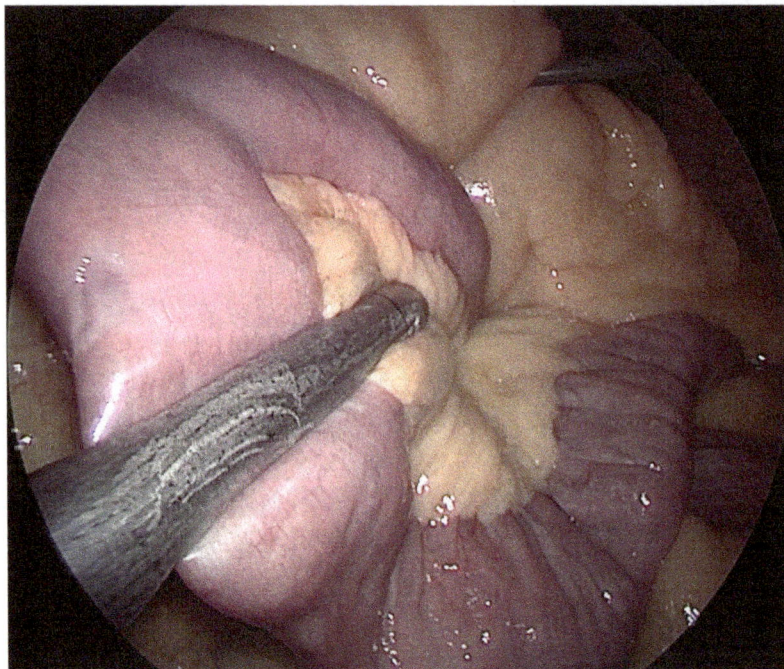

Figure 30. Transection of Bilio-pancreatic limb 20 cm from ligament of Treitz.

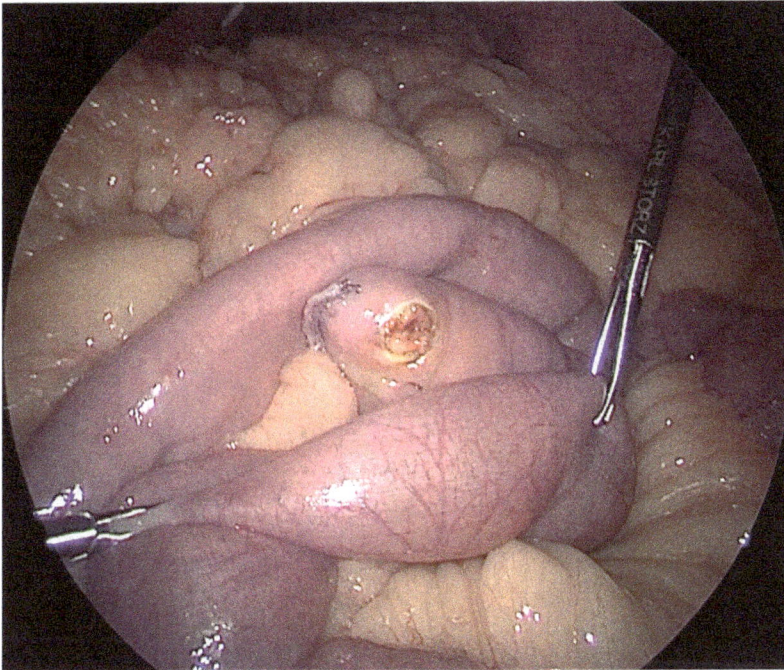

Figure 31. 300 cm bypassed proximal jejunum.

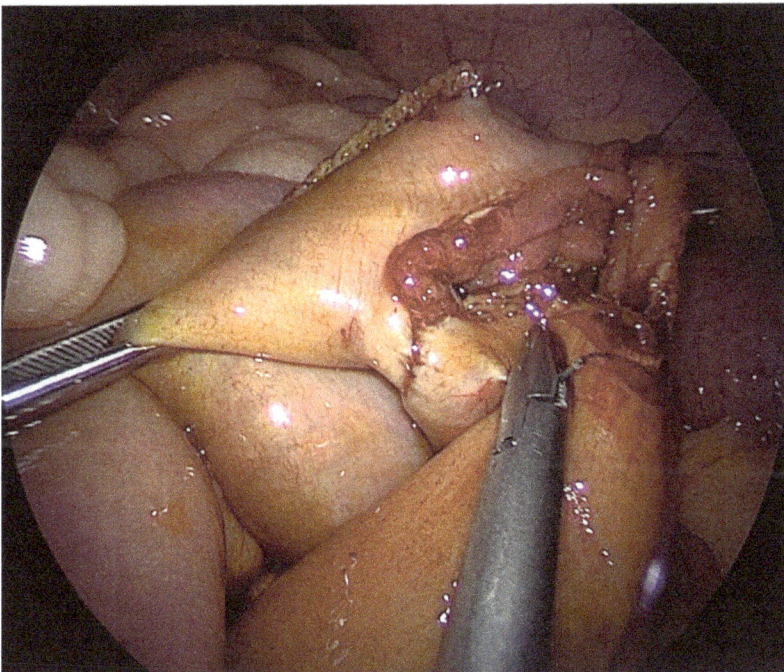

Figure 32. Closure of jejunojejunal anastomosis.

3.2.4.7. Gastric sleeve fixation

The suture line of the sleeved stomach is anchored with one or two stitches at the retroperitoneal fat using 3-0 Polyglactin 910 multifilament absorbable suture (J774D Ethicon 3-0 Coated Vicryl™ Taper SH). This prevents inadvertent twisting of the tubularized stomach (**Figure 33**).

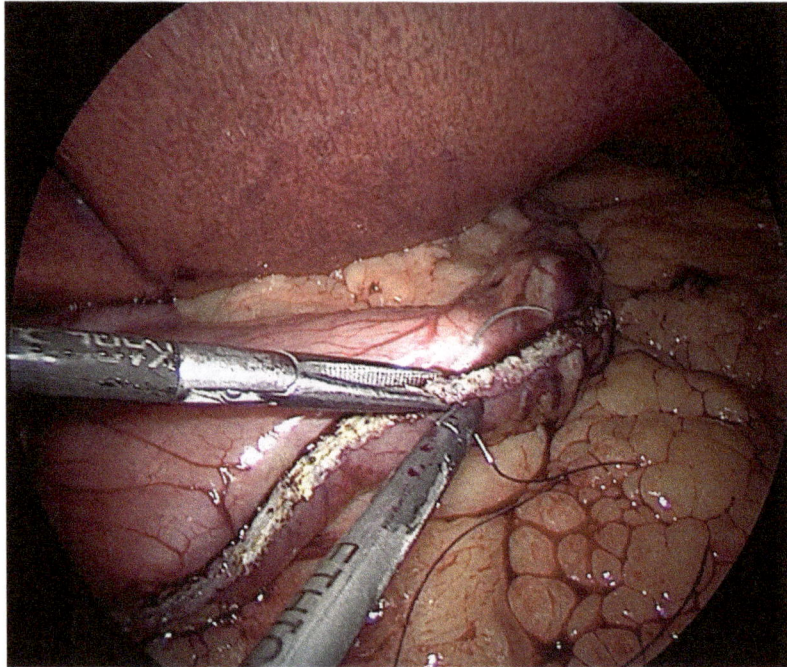

Figure 33. Anti torsion stitch.

3.2.5. Surgical Outcomes

Factors that contribute to the magnitude of weight loss and diabetic remission in sleeve-based procedures are still not fully elucidated. It probably owes its weight loss capabilities by eliminating the function of the stomach as a reservoir hereby reducing caloric content of processed food. Furthermore, because of the jejunojejunal bypass, the terminal ileum is exposed much earlier to undigested food and a more concentrated bile, both of which stimulate the release of incretins, primarily glucagon-like peptide 1 (GLP-1).

In the original study of Alamo et al., the average BMI and average weight at 12 months after vertical isolated gastroplasty with gastroenteral bypass were 23.4 ± 3.3 kg/m^2 (19.2–27.7) and 65.1 ± 15 kg (46–83) from 41.2 ± 5.1 kg/m^2 (35.3–57.8) and 110.7 ± 16.2 kg. The mean percent excess weight loss (% EWL) was $90.2 \pm 11.9\%$ [3]. In other studies, the mean BMI was reduced to 21.4 ± 1.9 kg/m^2 at 18 months' follow-up from 31.6 ± 2.1 kg/m^2 with a mean percent EWL of $75.7 \pm 8.5\%$. Comparing these figures with RYGB, in the study by Higa et al., where patients were followed-up for 10 years, the mean percent excess weight loss was 57% and the average postoperative BMI was 33 ± 8.0 kg/m^2 at 10 years [14].

In a cohort study of 49 patients (2012) evaluating the efficacy of SGPJB in ameliorating T2DM in patients with BMI < 35 kg/m^2, 81.6% (40/48) of patients with T2DM achieved complete remission after SGPJB with the remaining nine patients achieving improvement. As far as discontinuation of oral hyperglycemic agents and insulin dependence are concerned, 97.6% (40/41) of patients stopped taking their medications and 100% (8/8) stopped using insulin [10].

4. Laparoscopic Roux-En-Y Gastric Bypass (Figure 34)

Mason observed that distal gastrectomy with Billroth II reconstruction causes weight loss. The first open RYGB was performed for weight loss in 1967 while the first Laparoscopic RYGB was performed by Wittgrove [15]. Since then, laparoscopic RYGB is one of the most commonly performed bariatric procedure done for excess weight loss (**Figure 34**).

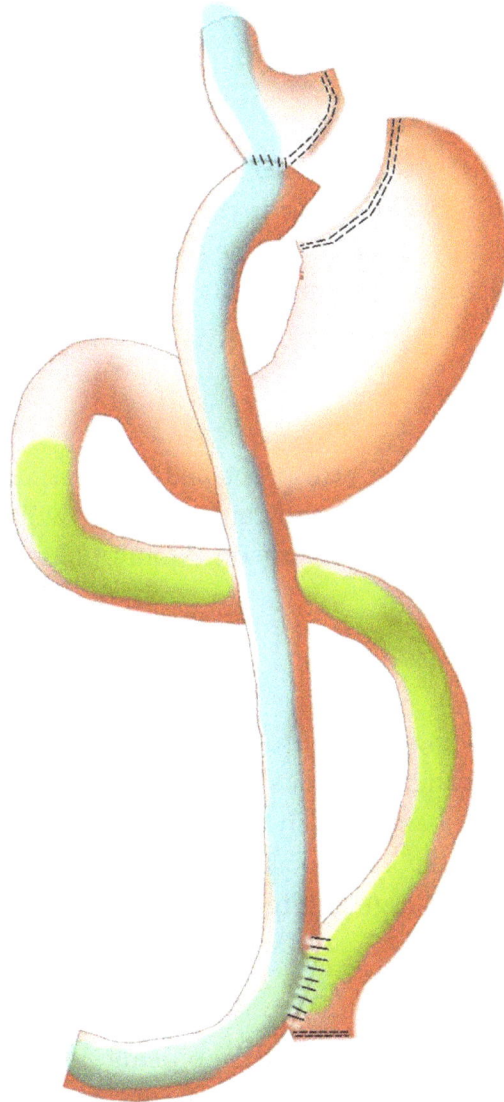

Figure 34. Schematic diagram of LRYGB.

Based on the 1991 NIH criteria, there are a number of widely accepted indication and contraindication which make a patient suitable for Bariatric or weight loss surgery:

- BMI > 40 without comorbidities.

- >35 with associated obesity-related illness such as diabetes or sleep apnea.

- Failed reasonable attempts at other weight loss techniques.

- Obesity-related health problems.

- No psychiatric or drug dependency problems.

- A capacity to understand the risks and commitment associated with surgery.

- Pregnancy not anticipated in the first 2 years following surgery.

For Asians, BMI is reduced by 2.5 for the above.

4.1. Operative technique

4.1.1. General preparations

Preoperative investigation includes standard basic blood profile, thyroid function test, serum cortisol level, HbA1c and C-peptide if diabetic, whole abdominal ultrasound and upper gastrointestinal endoscopy. Patient will be placed on NPO and started with intravenous drip 125–150 ml/h. Anticoagulants are usually not needed but thromboelastic stockings are applied.

4.1.2. Patient positioning

Patient is positioned supine with both arms stretched out. Surgeon will be on the right side of the patient while the assistant surgeon and camera holder will be on the left. The assisting nurse will stand on the same side as the surgeon. Monitor(s) are placed at the head end of patient.

4.1.3. Port placement

A 12 mm optical port placed 3-finger breadth left lateral to umbilicus. A 5 mm port is placed 4-finger breadth to the right of umbilicus for surgeons left hand working port. A 12 mm port is placed at 45 degrees to right hand port in the right mid clavicular line for surgeon's left hand and stapler insertion. Another 5 mm port is inserted in upper left subcostal region in the anterior axillary line for assistant surgeon (**Figure 35**).

4.1.4. Liver suspension tape

Liver retraction is done with liver suspension tape using a straight needle prolene suture-Jackson Pratt drain as previously described in this chapter for LSG.

4.1.5. Creation of gastric pouch

Gastric pouch is created by marking with orogastric calibration tube (OGCT) balloon with 25 ml insufflation. Perigastric dissection is done with hook diathermy at lesser curve with preservation of hepatic branch of vagus nerve, usually after the first vascular branch. Two-three staplers (medium thickness) are used to create the gastric pouch. The final pouch size would be about 15–20 ml. Adhesion on the posterior aspect of gastric pouch are cleared. A small gastrostomy is created at the posterior side of the pouch with hook diathermy for the creation of gastrojejunostomy (**Figures 36–42**).

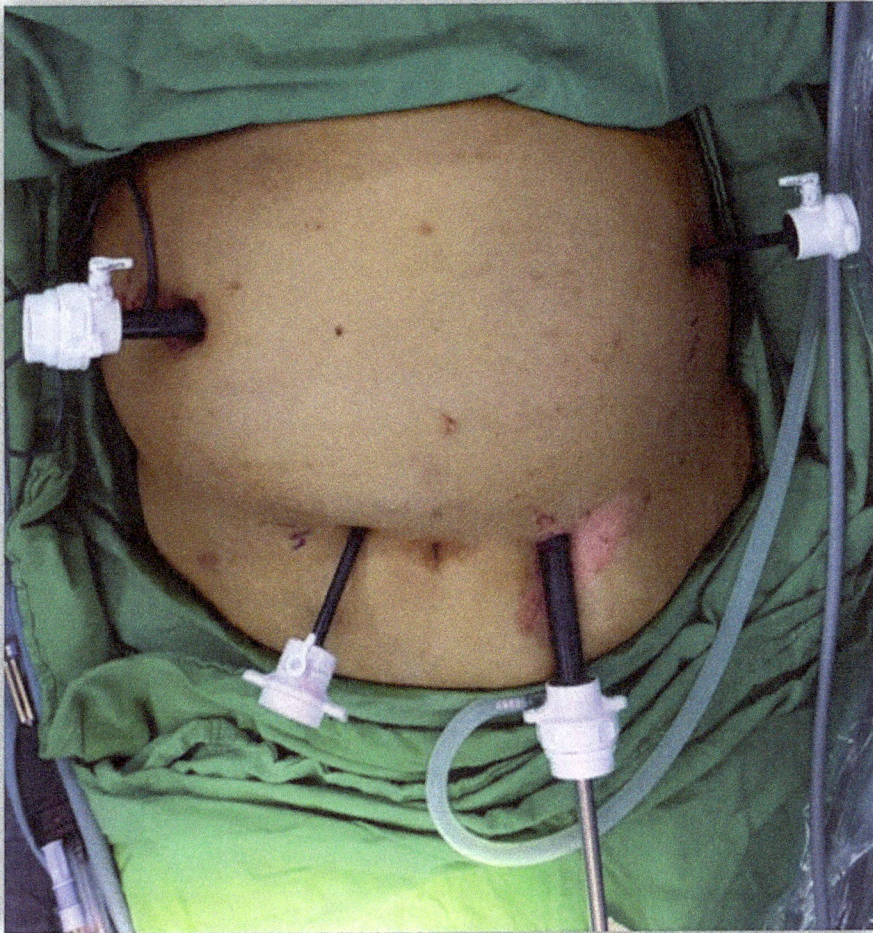

Figure 35. Port placement.

4.1.6. Gastrojejunostomy

Ligament of Treitz is identified and 100 cm of proximal jejunum is measured. Jejunotomy is created with hook cautery and loop of jejunum is anastomosed to the gastric pouch with linear stapler. Diameter of the gastrojejunal stoma is about 1.5–2 cm. Jejunum is disconnected just proximal to gastrojejunostomy with a 45 mm white cartridge reload (EGIA45AMT Endo GIA™ 45 mm articulating thin reload with Tri-Staple Technology or ECR45W Echelon Endopath™ tri-stapler reload cartridges by Ethicon) to avoid creating a "candy cane" blind loop. Closure of gastrojejunal enterotomy is performed with Monocryl 3-0. 38 Fr orogastric tube is passed through the gastrojejunal anastomosis to check for patency (**Figures 43–46**).

4.1.7. Jejunojejunostomy

Jejunum is measured for a distance of 100 cm from gastrojejunostomy and side to side jejunojejunostomy is created with 45 mm cartridge (EGIA45AMT Endo GIA™ 45 mm articulating thin reload with Tri-Staple Technology or ECR45W Echelon Endopath™ tri-stapler reload cartridges by Ethicon). Closure of jejunojejunal enterotomy is done with 3-0 Monocryl (**Figures 47** and **48**).

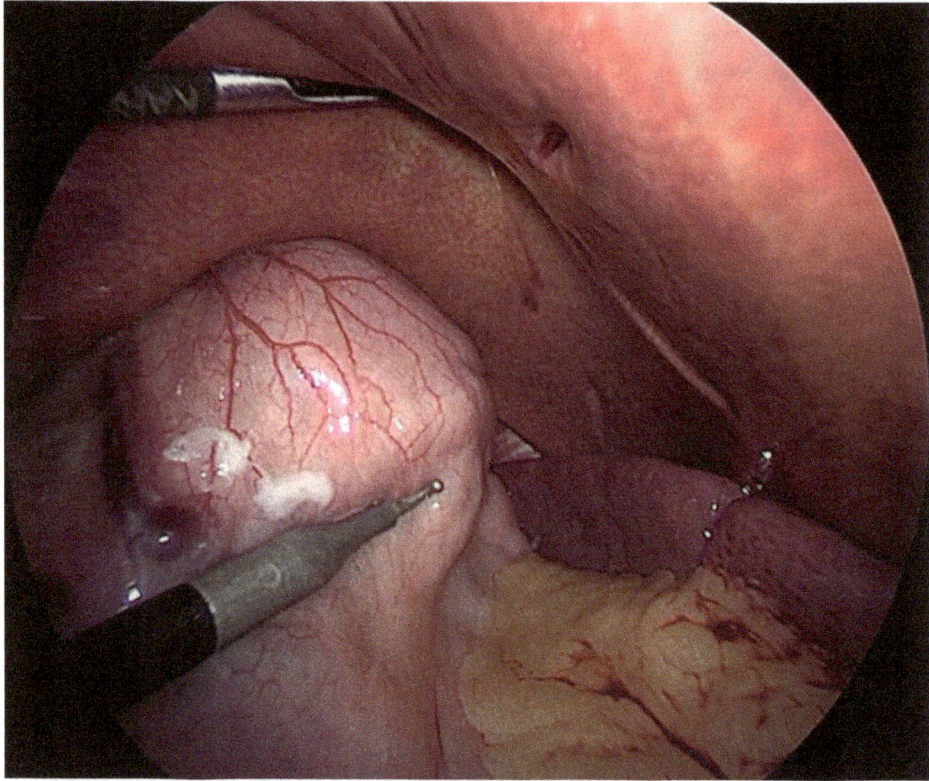

Figure 36. Calibration of gastric pouch.

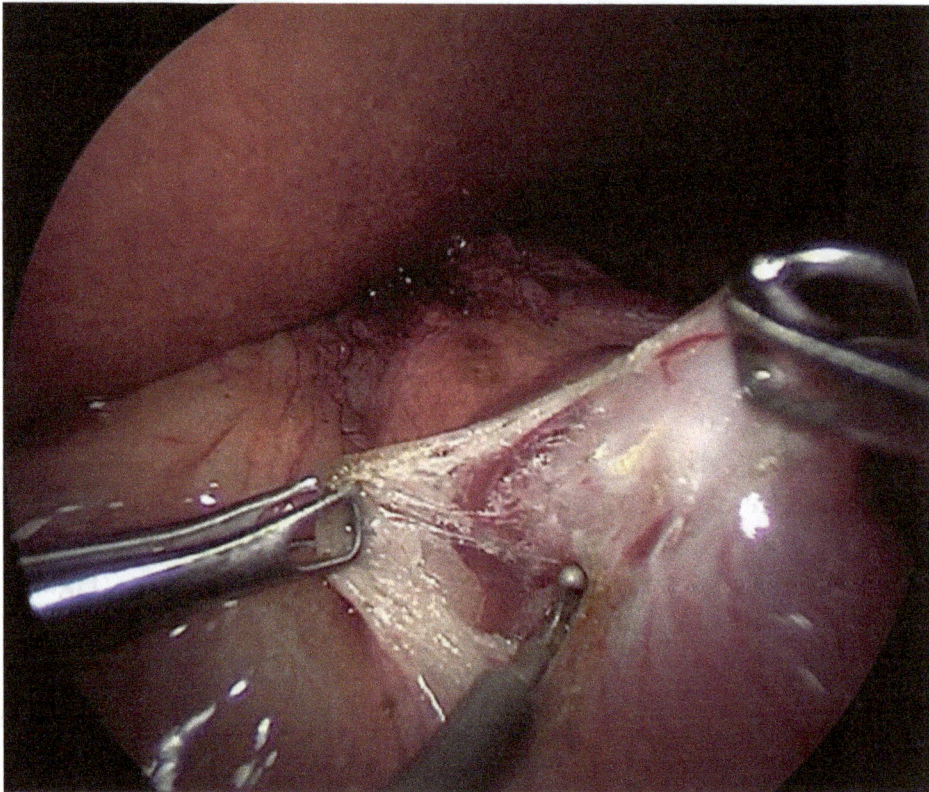

Figure 37. Perigastric dissection.

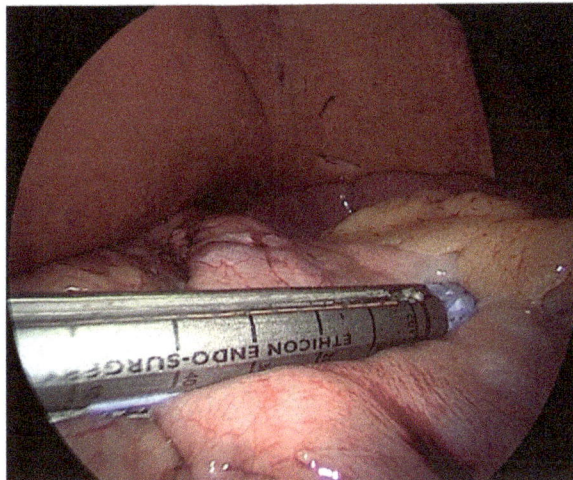

Figure 38. Firing of first staple.

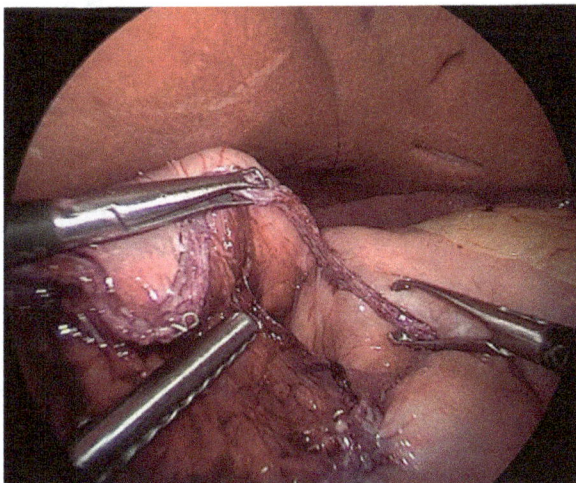

Figure 39. Dissection of adhesions at posterior gastric pouch.

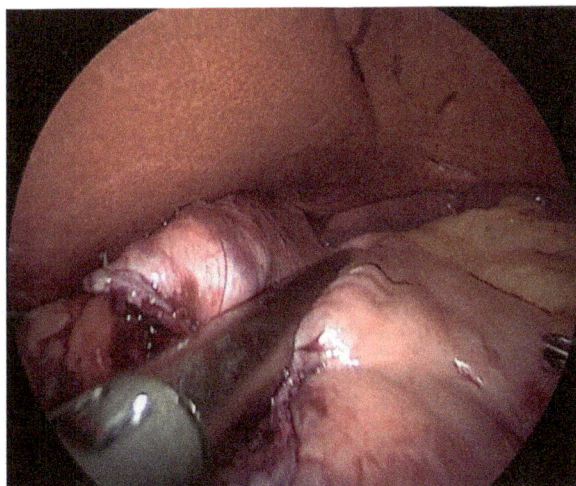

Figure 40. Firing of the 2nd stapler toward the angle of His.

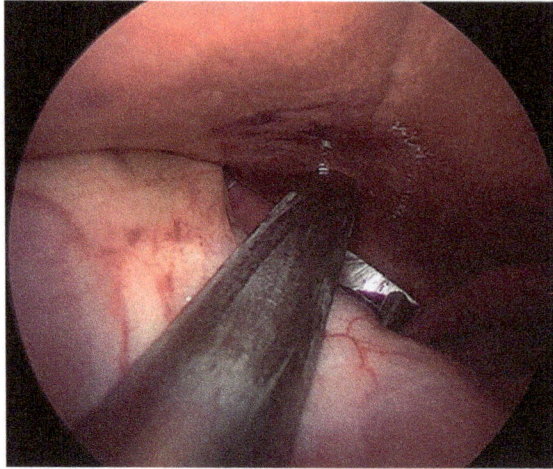

Figure 41. Firing of last stapler 1 cm away from GE junction.

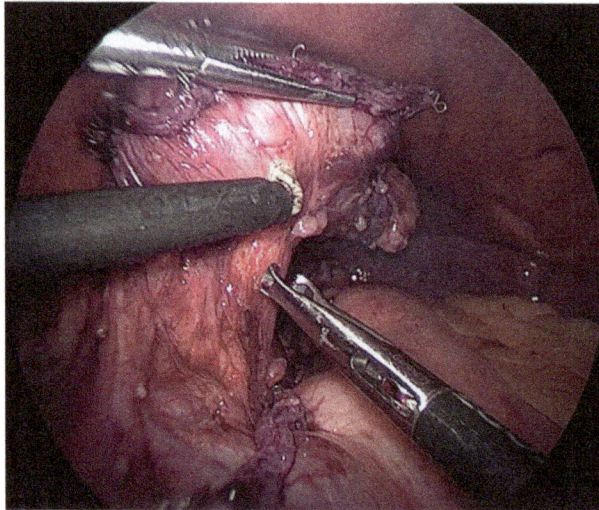

Figure 42. Creation of 1.5–2 cm gastrotomy.

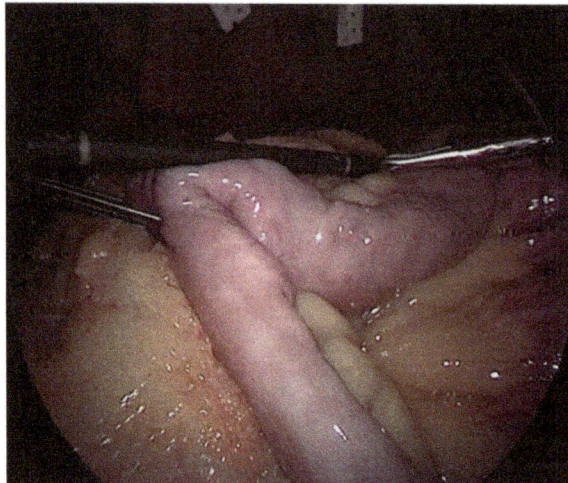

Figure 43. BP limb measuring 100–250 cm from the ligament of Treitz.

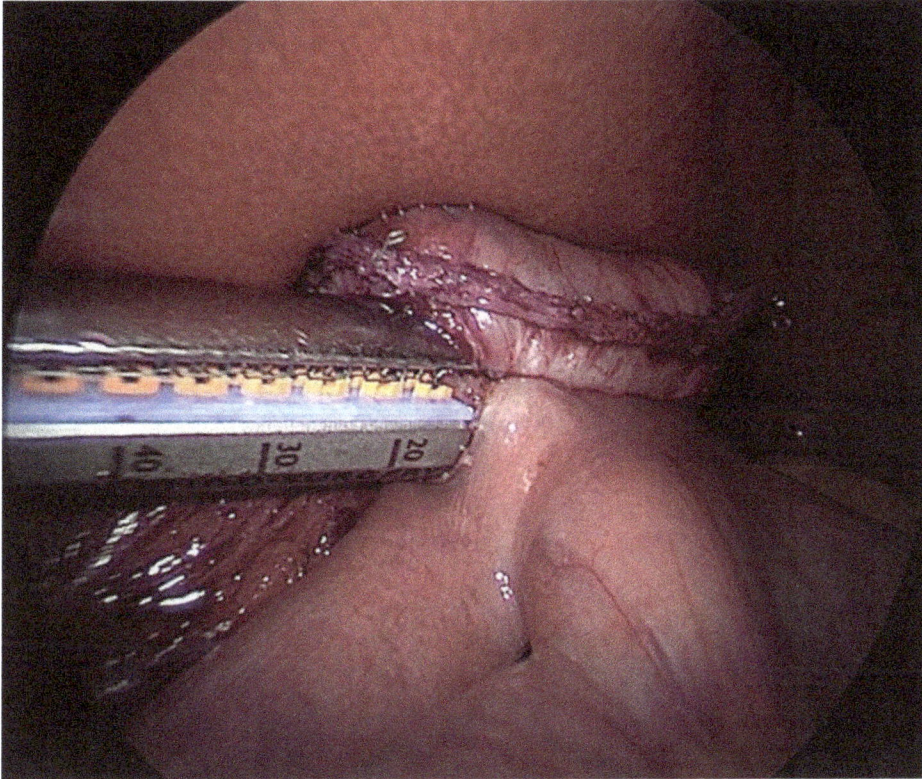

Figure 44. 1.5–2 cm side to side gastrojejunostomy.

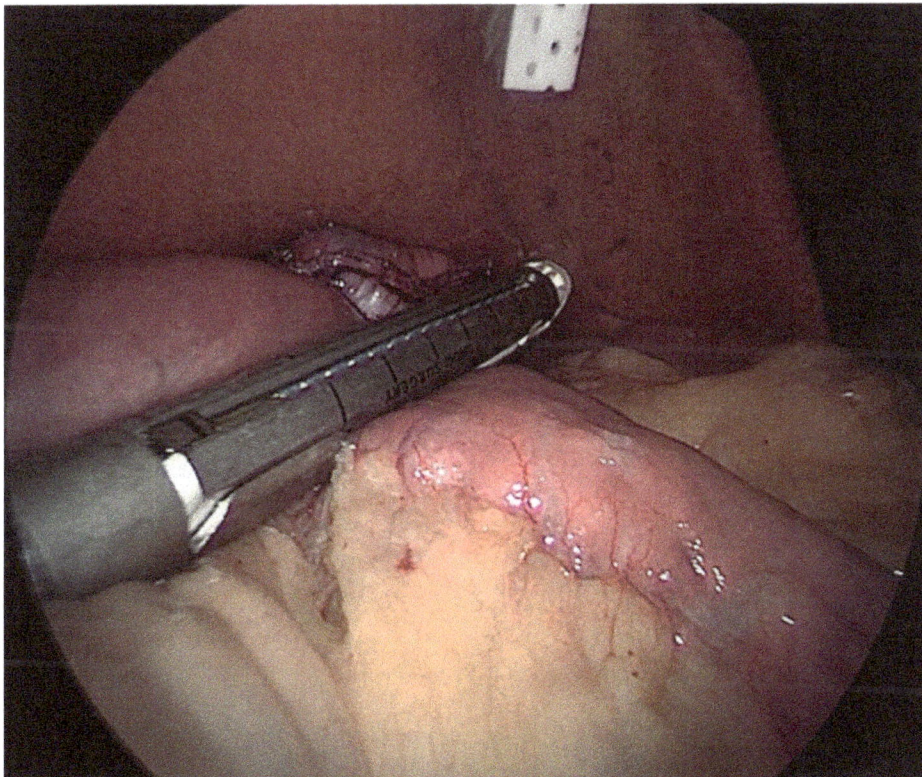

Figure 45. Transection of jejunum proximal to GJ anastomosis with thin stapler as close to GJ anastomosis as possible to avoid creating a candy cane stick blind loop.

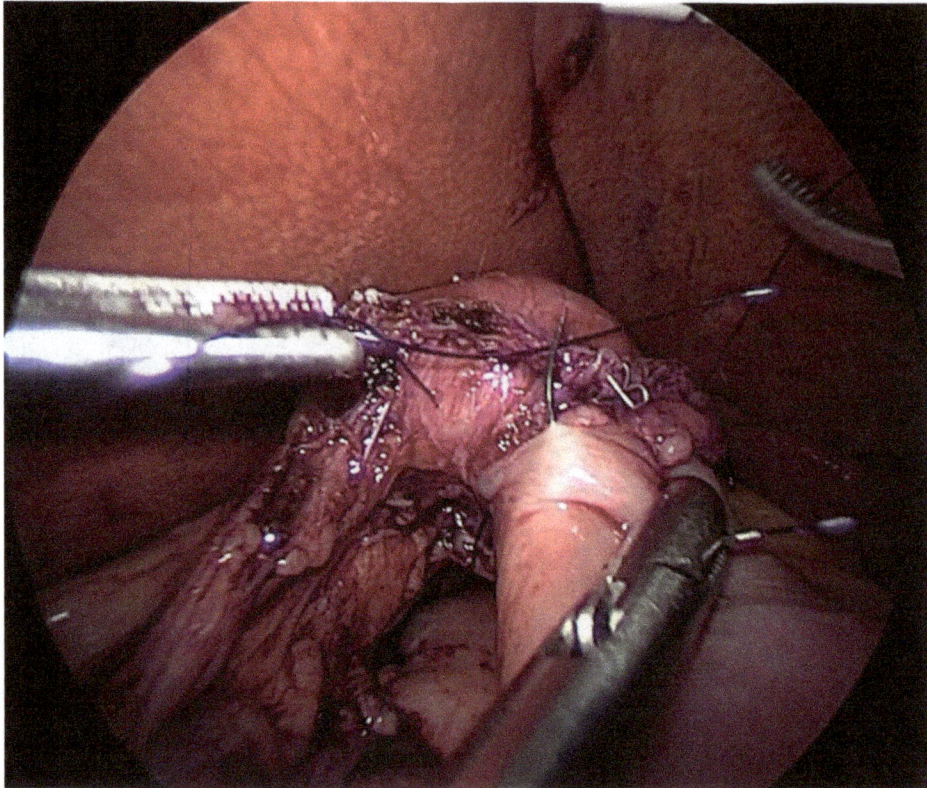

Figure 46. Gastrojejunal anastomosis completed by closure with single layer continuous suture using MONOSYN 3-0 round body needle.

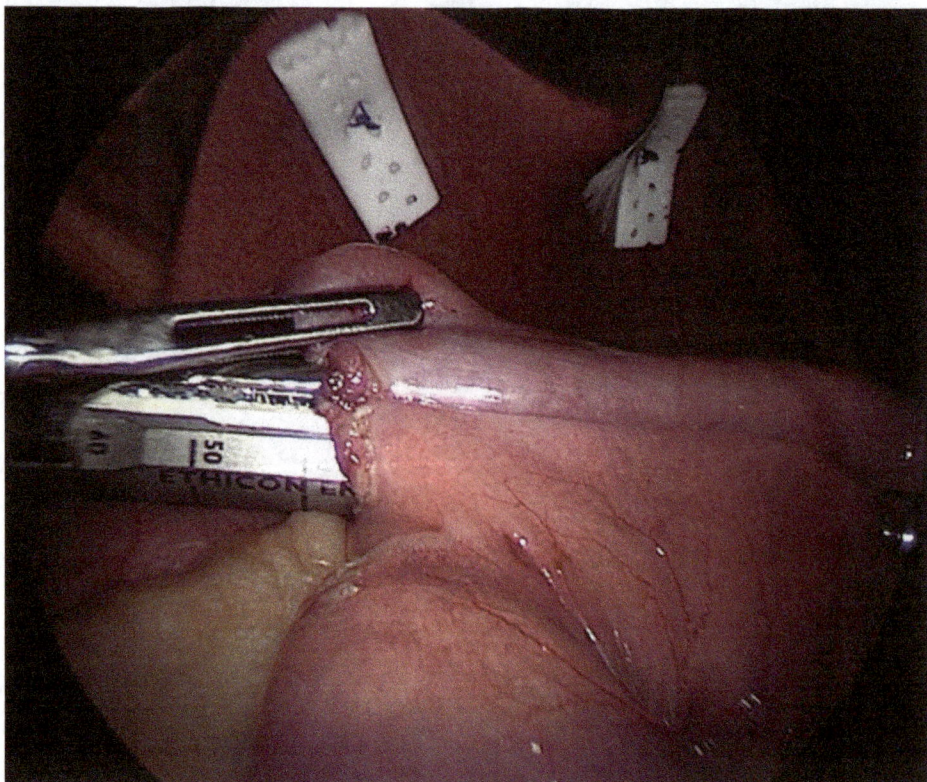

Figure 47. Side to side jejunojejunostomy.

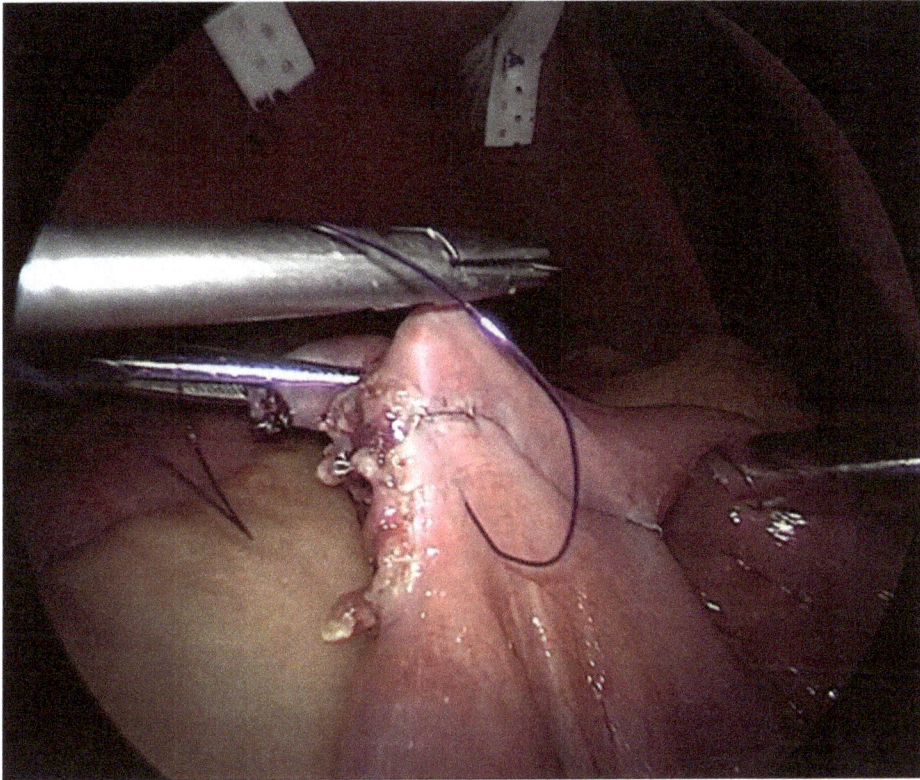

Figure 48. Hand-sewn closure of jejunojejunal anastomosis completed with single layer continuous suture using MONOSYN 3-0 round body needle.

4.1.8. Closure of mesenteric defects

Closure of mesenteric defects is performed with nonabsorbable sutures at jejunojejunal mesentery and Peterson defect (jejunotransverse mesocolon) to prevent internal herniation.

4.1.9. Removal of liver suspension, hemostasis, deflation and closure

After ensuring hemostasis at staple lines and anastomosis, liver suspension tapes are removed and hemostasis of liver punctures is done with diathermy.

4.2. Surgical outcome

4.2.1. Excess weight loss

Weight loss after bariatric surgery is dramatically seen in the first 12 months after surgery and continues at a slower rate up to 18 months postoperation. Excess weight loss after gastric bypass is between 72 and 82% within 12 months after surgery [16–18].

4.2.2. Improvement of comorbidities

Gastric bypass resulted in marked improvement in the biochemical markers of diabetes. Type 2 Diabetes Mellitus resolution is as high as 90.9% with mean fasting glucose reduction from 204 to 103 mg/dl, mean HbA1c reduction from 9.2 to 5.9% without T2DM medication in 12 months follow up. Up to 90% of patient did not need medication for control of glycaemia post operatively [19].

Gastric bypass can achieve a dramatic improvement of nonalcoholic fatty liver disease (NAFLD) both biochemically and histologically in morbid obesity [20]. Likewise, with significant weight loss and reduction of BMI after gastric bypass, pulmonary function improved in obese patients, which are correlated with decrease in waist circumference and possibly intra-abdominal pressure [21].

4.2.3. Complications

Complications occur in up to 20% patients and include anastomotic leak (0.25%), acute and late gastrojejuntostomy stricture (5%), gastrojejunostomy hemorrhage (1.5%), acute and late jejunojejunostomy stricture (1.5%), iron deficiency anemia, marginal ulcers hemorrhage (1.5%), gastric pouch dilatation (1.5%), nonspecific abdominal pain, hair loss, internal herniation if mesenteric defects are not closed and rarely peroneal nerve palsy, acute cholecystitis, biliary stone with obstruction and cholangitis and intra-abdominal abscess [16–18].

Author details

Chih Kun Huang[1]*, Sir Emmanuel S. Astudillo[2], Prasad M. Bhukebag[1] and Khan Wei Chan[1]

*Address all correspondence to: dr.ckhuang@hotmail.com

1 Body Science and Metabolic Disorders International (B.M.I.) Medical Center, China Medical University Hospital, Taichung City, Taiwan

2 Center for Diabetes, Nutrition & Weight Management, The Medical City Clark, Pampanga, Philippines

References

[1] Buchwald H, Avidor Y, Braunwald E, Jensen MD, Pories W, Fahrbach K, Schoelles K. Bariatric surgery: a systematic review and meta-analysis. JAMA. 2004;292(14):1724–1737.

[2] Rubino F, Nathan DM, Eckel RH, Schauer PR, Alberti KG, Zimmet PZ, Del Prato S, Ji L, Sadikot SM, Herman WH, Amiel SA, Kaplan LM, Taroncher-Oldenburg G, Cummings DE. Metabolic surgery in the treatment algorithm for type 2 diabetes: a joint statement by international diabetes organizations. Dia Care. 2016;39.6: 861–877. Web.

[3] Langer FB, Reza Hoda MA, Buhdjalian A, Felberbauer FX, Zacherl J, Wenzi E, Schindler K, Luger A, Ludvik B, Pregaer G. Sleeve gastrectomy and gastric banding: effects on plasma ghrelin levels. Obes Surg 2005;15(70):1024–1029.

[4] Himpens J, Dobbeleir J, Peeters G. Long-term results of laparoscopic sleeve gastrectomy for obesity. Ann Surg 2010;252 (2):319–324.

[5] Basso N, Leonetti F, Mariani P, et al. Early hormonal changes after sleeve gastrectomy in diabetic obese patients. Obes Surg. 2010;20(1):50–55.

[6]   Arman GA, Himpens J, Dhaenens J, et al. Long-term (11+years) outcomes in weight, patient satisfaction, comorbidities, and gastroesophageal reflux treatment after laparoscopic sleeve gastrectomy. Surg Obes Relat Dis 2016. [Epub ahead of print]. 10.1016/j. soard.2016.01.013

[7]   Huang CK, Goel R, Tai CM, et al. Novel metabolic surgery for type 2 diabetes mellitus: loop duodenojejunal bypass with sleeve gastrectomy. Surg Laparosc Endosc Percutan Tech 2013 Dec;23(6):481–485.

[8]   Huang CK, Ahluwalia JS, Garg A, Taweerutchana V, Ooi A, Chang PC, Hsin MC, et al. Novel Metabolic/Bariatric Surgery—Loop Duodenojejunal Bypass with Sleeve Gastrectomy (LDJB-SG). Essential and Controversies in Bariatric Surgery. 2014 Chapter 7: 133–144.

[9]   Alamo MA, Torres CS, Perez LZ, et al. Vertical isolated gastroplasty with gastro-enteral bypass: preliminary results. Obes Surg. 2006;16:353–358.

[10] Alamo M, Sepulveda M, Gellona J, Herrera M, Astorga C, Manterola C, et al. Sleeve gastrectomy with jejunal bypass for the treatment of type 2 diabetes mellitus in patients with body mass index <35 kg/m^2: a cohort study. Obes Surg. 2012;22:1097–1103.

[11] Huang CK, Tai CM, Chang PC, Malapan K, Tsai CC, Yolsuriyanwong K et al. Loop duodenojejunal bypass with sleeve gastrectomy: comparative study with Roux-en-Y gastric bypass in type 2 diabetic patients with a BMI <35 kg/m^2, first year results. Obes Surg. 2016;26(10):1–11.

[12] Lee WJ, Lee KT, Kasama K, Seike Y, Ser KH, Chun SC, Chen JC, Lee YC, et al. Laparoscopic single-anastomosis duodenal–jejunal bypass with sleeve gastrectomy (SADJB-SG): short-term result and comparison with gastric bypass. Obes Surg. 2014;24:109–113.

[13] Lee WJ, Almulai AM, Tsou JJ, Ser KH, Lee YC, Chen SC, et al. Duodenal–jejunal bypass with sleeve gastrectomy versus the sleeve gastrectomy procedure alone: the role of duodenal exclusion. Surg Obes Relat Dis. 2015 Jul–Aug; 11(4):765–770.

[14] Higa K, Ho T, Tercero F, Yunus, T, Boone K, et al. Laparoscopic Roux-en-Y gastric bypass: 10-year follow-up. Surg Obes Relat Dis. 2011;7:516–525.

[15] Wittgrove, et al. Laparoscopic gastric bypass, Roux-en-Y: preliminary report of 5 cases. Obes Surg. 1994;4:353–357.

[16] Huang, et al. Laparoscopic Roux-en-Y gastric bypass for morbidly obese Chinese patients: learning curve, advocacy and complications. Obes J. 2008; 18:776–781.

[17] Huang, et al. Use of individual surgeon versus surgical team approach: surgical team outcomes of laparoscopic Roux-en-Y gastric bypass in an Asian medical center. Surg Obes Relat Dis. 2012;8:214–219.

[18] Sjostrom L. Review of the key results from the Swedish obese subjects (SOS) trial— a prospective controlled intervention study of bariatric surgery. J Inter Med. 2013; 273(3):219–34.

[19] Huang, et al. Laparoscopic Roux-en-Y gastric bypass for the treatment of Type II diabetes mellitus in Chinese patients with body mass index of 25–35. Obes Surg. 2011;21:1344–1349.

[20] Tai et al. Improvement of non-alcoholic fatty liver disease after bariatric surgery in morbidly obese Chinese patients. Obes Surg. 2012;22:1016–1021.

[21] Wei, et al. Surgically induced weight loss, including reduction in waist circumference, is associated with improved pulmonary function in obese patients. Surg Obes Relat Dis. 2011;7:599–604.

8

Robotic Hysterectomy for Cancer and Benign Pathology

Adrian Kohut, Leah Goldberg and
Alexandre Buckley De Meritens

Abstract

The da Vinci Surgical System is an innovative technology that has advanced the laparoscopic treatment of benign and malignant diseases in gynecology. In this chapter, we will discuss the da Vinci Surgical System technology, including its history, utilization, surgical technique for benign and oncologic hysterectomy, future directions and surgical complications. Through a review of the literature, we aim to chronicle the current trends of application in both benign and oncologic gynecologic conditions and describe the current standards of care in this innovative and evolving operative technology. Although the future utility of robotic surgeries and robotic hysterectomies necessitates further research, the potential application of this surgical method affords great promise.

Keywords: robotic hysterectomy, gynecologic oncology, benign gynecologic surgery

1. History

The initial da Vinci robotic surgical system (Intuitive Surgical, Sunnyvale, CA) was released in Europe in 1999 and received FDA approval in 2000 [1]. In 2005, the FDA approved the da Vinci robotic system for gynecological surgeries. The first system consisted of two robotic operating arms and one camera holder. Since its emergence in the surgical arena, there have been four updates to the system, each of which has increased its overall capability within various surgical subspecialties and overall maneuverability of instrument use. The latest version termed the da Vinci Xi was released in 2014 and includes 3D HD vision, four quadrant mounting, and instruments capable of moving in seven degrees of motion while performing complex surgical techniques including clamping, cutting, coagulating, dissecting, suturing and manipulating tissue [2].

In 2002, Diaz-Arrastia et al. published a series of 11 patients undergoing uncomplicated da Vinci assisted total laparoscopic hysterectomy and bilateral salpingo-oophorectomy demonstrating feasibility for its use in gynecologic surgery [3]. Subsequently, Lambaudie et al. published a report of 28 patients undergoing various da Vinci assisted surgical procedures for gynecologic cancer including total hysterectomy, bilateral oophorectomy, and pelvic and/or para-aortic lymphadenectomy. The authors found that the use of robot-assisted laparoscopy led to less intraoperative blood loss, less postoperative pain and shorter hospital stays compared with those treated with more traditional surgical approaches such as laparoscopy and laparotomy [4]. The following year the FDA approved the use of the da Vinci robotic system for use in gynecologic oncology surgery.

2. Introduction

Over the past 12 years, the da Vinci assisted approach to laparoscopic hysterectomy has taken a more prominent role in the surgical management of a multitude of benign and oncologic gynecologic conditions. Multiple meta-analyses and literature reviews have shown that the use of robotic surgery offers the advantage of decreased blood loss and length of stay when compared to open surgical techniques [5]. When compared to traditional laparoscopic methods outcomes appear to be equivocal, but a case can be made for the advantages of robotic surgery to treat obese patients [6]. The main disadvantages of robotic gynecologic surgery include increased intraoperative time and cost-effectiveness questionability. Such issues may be mitigated as operator proficiency increases. Future projections of advancement in robotic gynecologic surgery highlight the use of minimal incisions and single site approaches [7].

Hysterectomy is one of the most frequently performed surgical procedures in the United States. Common benign indications include symptomatic uterine leiomyomas (51.4%), abnormal uterine bleeding (41.7%), endometriosis (30%), and prolapse (18.2%) [8, 9].

The American College of Obstetricians and Gynecologists favors vaginal hysterectomy as the preferred method among women undergoing hysterectomy for benign disease [10]. A 2015 Cochrane Database Systematic Review indicated that vaginal hysterectomy appears to be superior to both laparoscopic hysterectomy and abdominal hysterectomy as it is associated with faster return to normal activities [11]. However, in cases involving factors such as adnexal pathology, severe endometriosis, adhesions, or an enlarged uterus, vaginal hysterectomy may not be appropriate [10]. Compared to abdominal hysterectomy, laparoscopic hysterectomy is associated with decreased risk of perioperative complications, faster return to normal activity, decreased length of hospital stay, decreased risk of readmission, decreased risk of surgical site infection, decreased blood loss and need for blood transfusion, and improved postoperative quality of life [11]. Though current evidence demonstrates a less significant difference between robot-assisted laparoscopic hysterectomy and conventional laparoscopic hysterectomy, potential benefits of the robotic-assisted approach include decreased complication rate, decreased length of hospital stay, decreased blood loss and need for blood transfusion, and decreased risk of conversion to exploratory laparotomy for surgically complicated cases and obese patients [9, 12–19]. With an increasing number of both academic institutions and community hospitals offering robotic surgery, there is a national uptrend in rates of the robotic-assisted approach. Of all benign hysterectomies, robotic-assisted surgery increased from 0.5% in 2007 to 9.5% in 2010 [9, 13, 18, 20–27].

In the context of gynecologic oncology, common indications for hysterectomy include cancers of the endometrium, cervix, ovary or fallopian tube. The 2017 NCCN Clinical Practice Guidelines in Oncology for Uterine Neoplasm state that "Minimally invasive hysterectomy is now the preferred approach when technically feasible" [28]. The randomized controlled trial LAP2 showed short-term surgical benefits of laparoscopy over laparotomy for uterine cancer staging, and follow-up data showed equivalent oncologic outcomes [29]. In the case of cervical cancer, even though we do not have phase III data supporting the use of minimally invasive surgery, there is a body of literature demonstrating feasibility and suggesting equivalent oncologic outcomes compared to abdominal hysterectomy [30–32].

Robotic surgery has taken center stage in becoming the standard of care in patients with early-stage endometrial and cervical cancer. When comparing robotic-assisted surgery with conventional laparoscopy for endometrial cancer, robotic surgery has been found to have decreased length of stay, reduced operating time, decreased blood loss, and more rapid postsurgical recovery [6]. Furthermore, robotic surgery has even been shown to result in high lymph note count as compared to conventional laparoscopy when performed in obese women with endometrial cancer [33]. In comparing robot-assisted surgery with abdominal surgery for endometrial cancer, robotic surgery is associated with decreased blood loss, reduced length of stay, increased operation duration, and equal number of lymph node counts [20, 34–40]. In analyzing total cost of care for endometrial cancer patients, robotic surgery has been shown to be significantly cheaper ($8212.00 versus $12,943.60, P = .001) due to its association with a decreased length of stay [20, 34, 41]. In patients with early cervical cancer, robotic-assisted and conventional laparoscopic radical hysterectomy have both been shown to be superior to exploratory laparotomy due to decreased blood loss, decreased complication rates, reduced the length of stay, and increased lymph node count. In such patients, there is conflicting data showing the advantage of the robotic approach over conventional laparoscopy [36, 42–58]. There is currently limited data on the use of robotics in the setting of advanced ovarian cancer, and thus its use is not recommended at this time [3, 4, 59–63].

In this chapter, we will describe the technology behind the robotic-assisted surgery, patient preparation, surgical technique for simple and radical hysterectomy and complications.

3. The technology

Robot-assisted laparoscopy is an innovative advancement in gynecologic laparoscopic surgery. The robotic approach enhances traditional laparoscopy by providing three-dimensional optics, advanced ergonomics, improved vision and precision, tremor filtration, and 7° of motion with advanced dexterity [2]. There are currently four generations of the da Vinci Surgical System: The "standard", the S, the Si, the X and the Xi system. The components of the da Vinci Surgical System include the surgeon console, the patient side cart, and the vision system [2] (**Figure 1**).

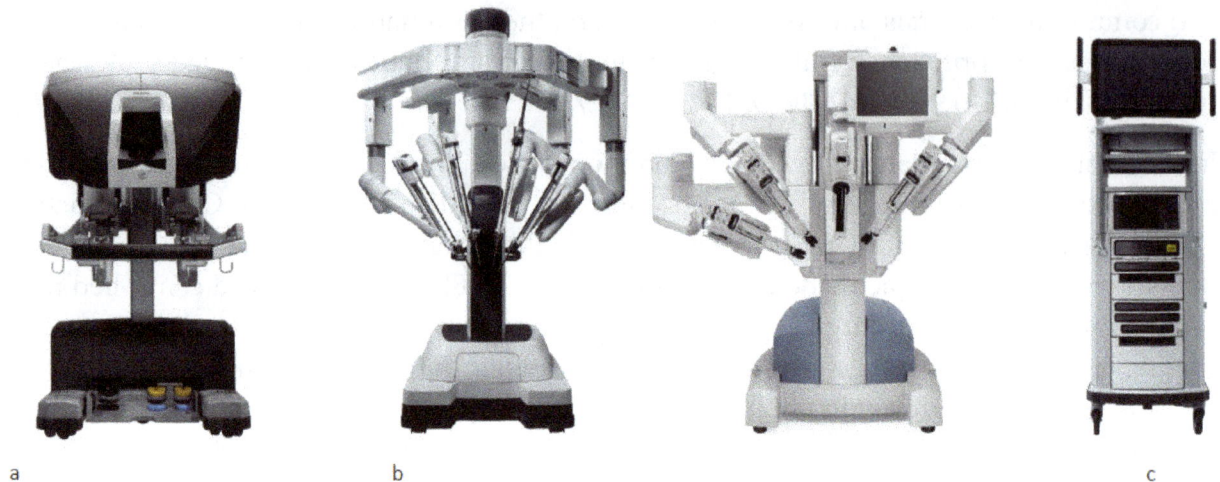

a   b   c

Figure 1. (a) Surgeons console; (b) patients side-cart; and (c) vision tower.

The surgeon operates seated at the console while viewing a 3D high-definition image inside the patient's body. The surgeon's fingers grasp the master controls below the display which converts the surgeon's hand, wrist and finger movements into precise, simultaneous movements of surgical instruments [2].

The patient-side cart is where the patient is positioned during surgery. Attached to the side cart are four robotic arms that facilitate the surgeon's commands by moving around fixed pivot points which allow for less force on the abdominal wall than laparoscopy [2]. The vision system is equipped with a 3D, high-definition endoscope and image processing equipment for visualization of the patient's anatomy [2]. A view of the operating field is available to the entire OR team on a large viewing monitor (vision cart) [2].

A full range of EndoWrist instruments (Intuitive Surgical, Sunnyvale, CA) is available to the surgeon while operating. Most instruments are modeled after the human wrist, offering a greater range of motion than the human hand. Each instrument is designed for a particular task, such as clamping, cutting, coagulating, dissecting, suturing and manipulating tissue. EndoWrist Instruments feature 7° of freedom, 90° of articulation, natural motion and finger-tip control, motion scaling and tremor reduction [2]. Energy instruments include da Vinci monopolar and bipolar cautery instruments (electrical energy), the da Vinci Harmonic™ ACE (mechanical energy), the da Vinci PK™ Dissecting Forceps (advanced bipolar), and laser [2]. Grasping instruments allow handling thin, delicate tissues as well as thicker and stronger tissues. Needle drivers provide the ability to suture with fine and thick needles. SutureCut™ Needle Drivers include a cutting blade for efficient cutting of suture after knot tying [2].

4. Indications

Robotic hysterectomy may be employed for a wide spectrum of benign pathologies including leiomyoma, abnormal uterine bleeding, endometriosis, adenomyosis, adnexal mass, pelvic pain, and pelvic organ prolapse. Common malignant pathologies necessitating hysterectomy include primary cancers of the uterus, ovary, cervix, fallopian tubes, and peritoneum; as well as nongynecologic metastases of urologic, colorectal, breast, gastrointestinal, renal, pulmonary, melanomatous, or lymphatic origin.

5. Technique

After induction of general endotracheal anesthesia and insertion of an orogastric tube, the patient is placed in dorsal lithotomy position using yellowfin stirrups with careful padding of pressure points. Both arms are padded and tucked to the sides. The patient is placed in steep Trendelenburg position (27–30°) to allow mobilization of the small bowel out the pelvic area and exposing the aorta if in need to perform lymph node dissection. She is prepped and draped in the standard sterile fashion. Foley catheter is inserted, and a uterine manipulator such as a V-care manipulator (ConMed Endosurgery, Utica, NY) or the Advincula Arch uterine manipulator (Cooper Surgical, Trumbull, CT) is placed. The uterine manipulator allows demarcation of the cervicovaginal junction necessary to perform the colpotomy.

5.1. Port placement

Port placement can differ based on uterine size, the need to do lymph node dissection, using 2 or 3 operative arms and the da Vinci system used (**Figure 2**). The endoscope port is the reference port for all other ports. If not doing lymph node dissection and with a small uterus, the camera port can be placed 8–10 cm above the fundus which ends up being at the umbilicus. For oncologic surgery, we place the camera port 20–25 cm above the pubic bone [64]. When using the S or Si system we place a 10–12 mm laparoscopic port for the camera and when using the Xi system we place the 8 mm da Vinci camera trocar. The ports need to be 6–10 cm apart to allow triangulation and avoid arms collision. When using three operative arms, the surgeon can decide to place the third arm either at the right or left hemi-abdomen. Placing the third operative arm on the right will result in controlling both arms with the surgeon's right hand and vice versa if placed on the left hemi-abdomen.

When using the Xi system the operative ports can be placed in a straight line at the level of the umbilicus but all ports can be shifted up for a large uterus or for lymph node dissection. The assist port is usually placed 2–3 cm under the left rib cage over the mid-clavicular line (Palmer point) but can be place in the lower quadrants. Careful placement should be done to avoid placing the assistant port in a straight line with the target anatomy and an operative port. This would result in difficult access to the surgical field for the assistant. We like using either a 5 or 8 mm Airseal trocar for the assist port (ConMed Utica, NY). When using the S or Si systems operative ports should be placed 8–10 cm apart and keeping 10–20 cm distance to the target anatomy.

5.2. Docking the patient-side cart

For gynecologic surgery, docking can be done either between the patient's legs or from the side (**Figure 3**). We like side docking because it allows for an assistant to occupy the space between

a.

Initial endoscope port at the umbilicus

b.

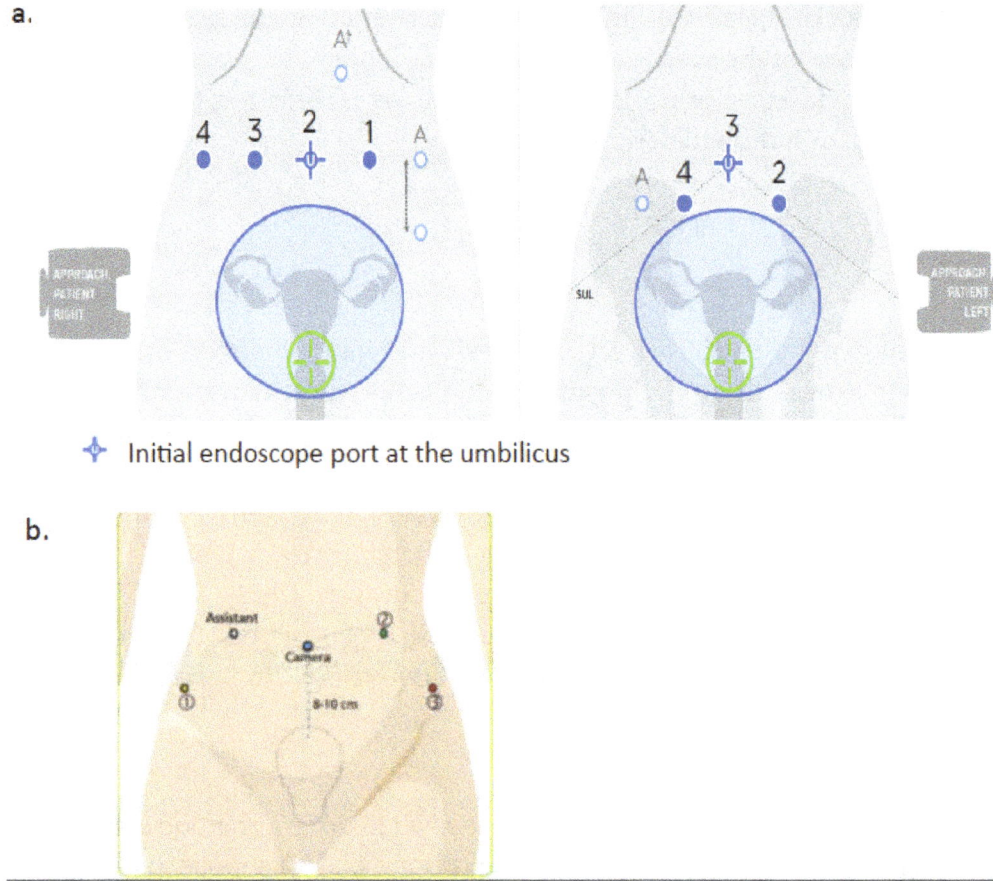

Figure 2. (a) Port placement for the Xi system showing 3 operative arms and 2 operative arms configuration and (b) port placement for the S and Si systems.

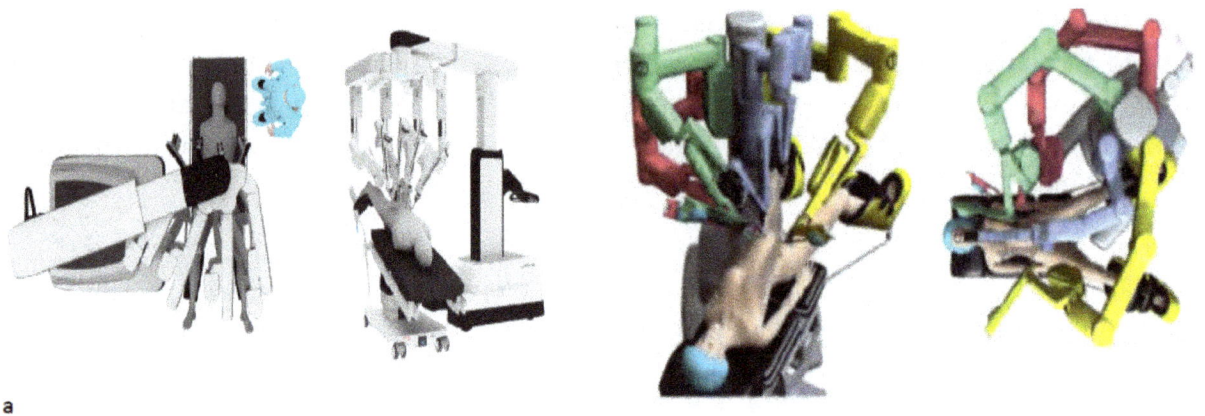

a

Figure 3. Side docking. Side docking with the Xi and S system.

the legs and use the uterine manipulator and deliver specimens through the vagina without difficulty. When using the S system, the robotic column is positioned at a 45° acute angle relative to the cephalad/caudal axis of the patient. When using the Xi system the patient-side cart can be approached in almost any angle to the bed and the arms are rotated to fix their position.

5.3. Simple hysterectomy technique

A survey of the entire abdominal cavity is performed laparoscopically. Once the robotic column is successfully docked bipolar forceps are inserted into the left-sided instrument port, monopolar scissors are inserted into the right-sided instrument port, and a grasper inserted into the rightmost port. The assistant seated at the left upper quadrant assistant port starts the procedure with a suction irrigator, laparoscopic bowel grasper, laparoscopic Maryland, and laparoscopic scissors all on hand.

The pelvic peritoneum is incised parallel to the infundibulopelvic ligament. The external iliac artery is identified and traced down to the bifurcation of the common iliac artery. The ureter is found entering the pelvis at the level of the bifurcation. At this point, the ovarian vessels contained in the infundibulopelvic ligament are isolated from the ureter by creating a window in the posterior sheet of the broad ligament. Either the ovarian vessels are clamped, cauterized and transected if a salpingo-oophorectomy is intended or the utero-ovarian ligament. The posterior sheet of the broad ligament is extended in the direction of the uterosacral ligament skeletonizing the uterine artery. The round ligament is then clamped, cauterized and transected. The anterior sheet of the broad ligament is opened in the direction of the vesicouterine peritoneal reflexion. After performing this procedure bilaterally, the bladder is mobilized off of the upper vagina to expose the cervicovaginal junction marked by the colpotomizer of the uterine manipulator. The uterine vessels are then clamped, cauterized and transected at a 90° angle at the cervico-uterine junction. The cardinal ligament is then clamped, cauterized and transected medially to the uterine vessel pedicle and parallel to the cervix. After performing the colpotomy, the specimen is delivered through the vagina. A sterile glove filled with a lap sponge is inserted into the vagina once the specimen is successfully extracted to maintain adequate pneumoperitoneum. The vaginal cuff is then closed using either one polysorb or v-lock suture.

5.4. Radical hysterectomy

The surgical technique is similar to the traditional Type III abdominal radical hysterectomy. The avascular spaces (pararectal, paravesical and obturator spaces) are developed to identify the ureters, the major vessels (external and interior iliac arteries, the superior vesical and uterine arteries), the obturator nerve and the genitofemoral nerve (**Figure 4**). The uterine artery is cauterized and transected at its origin and mobilized medially to expose the ureter. Complete ureterolysis is performed to the canal of Wertheim, and the ureter is then unroofed allowing to mobilize both the ureter and the bladder away from the upper third of the vagina. The peritoneum between both uterosacral ligaments is incised, and the paravesical space is bluntly developed, thus allowing transection of the uterosacral ligament at its origin. The paracolpos is then clamped, cauterized and transected parallel to the vagina allowing to perform the upper vaginectomy.

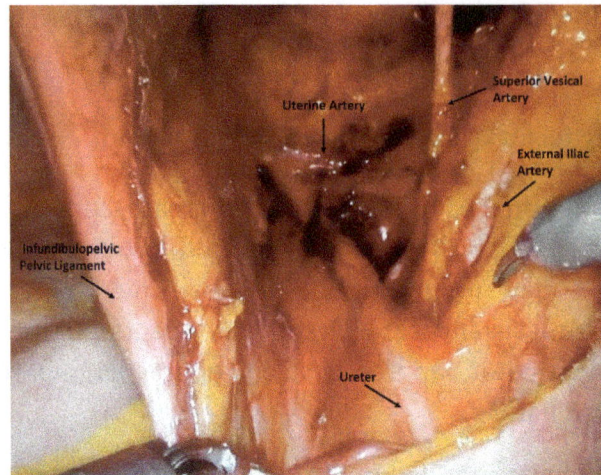

Figure 4. Right retroperitoneal pelvic sidewall anatomy.

6. Future robotic surgery

6.1. Multiport and single port

Single port laparoscopy is a relatively new advancement in minimally invasive surgery. Da Vinci surgery with Single-Site has been approved for cholecystectomy, hysterectomy, and salpingo-oophorectomy in benign conditions. Traditional or robotic-assisted single port laparoscopy for hysterectomy and other gynecologic procedures such as myomectomy and adnexal surgery has been reported in the literature with favorable outcomes [65–67]. Known advantages include improved cosmetic appearance as there is only one incision, decrease postoperative pain and wound infection, and minimization of potential damage to vasculature during port placement [68, 69]. However, single port laparoscopy has technical difficulties including instrument crowding leading to increased collision between instruments and limited degree of movement. There is also an increased risk of an incision-site hernia with single-port surgery. The da Vinci with Single-site technology for a hysterectomy requires a multichannel access port with an insufflation valve and space for four cannulas. Two curved ports are for the robotic controlled instruments, one port holds the endoscope, and the final one is the designated assistant port. In the current literature, there are only retrospective study designs that compare single port laparoscopy with multiport while using the da Vinci robotic system. Paek et al. compared surgical outcomes of single robotic site (n = 25) and laparoendoscopic single-site total hysterectomy (n = 442) for benign disease states [70]. The study found that the robotic group had a lower complication rate, and less operative bleeding, however, there was significantly longer operating times when compared to the laparoscopic group. Lopez et al. also found an increase in total operative time (approximately 25 min) while using the robotic-assisted single site compared to laparoscopic single site [71]. In this study, there was a significant decrease in length of hospital stay by 8 h in the robotic arm. Gungor et al. compared the operative time, perioperative and early operative complication rate, conversion to another technique rate, postoperative pain, and recovery time, and found that there were no significant differences between single site laparoscopy vs. robotic hysterectomy for benign disease [72]. Single site robotic and laparoscopic surgery was deemed to be safe and feasible techniques for total hysterectomy. In the hands of an experienced robotic surgeon, the learning curve of robotic laparoendoscopic single site surgery is fast, requiring 13 cases significantly decrease operative time [73]. While single port robotic-assisted hysterectomy seems promising, a Cochrane review reports that there is a lack of evidence of any benefit of a single port or robot-assisted hysterectomy when compared to traditional multi-port laparoscopic hysterectomy [11]. Future randomized control trials are needed to evaluate the potential advantages of robotic single site surgery.

7. Surgical complications

New causes of complication have been introduced with robotic-assisted surgery, but the overall incidence of complications is similar to those of conventional laparoscopic surgery. The FDA database reports 21% of injuries attributed to operator-related error and 14% to technical system failure [74]. The main drawback from robotic-assisted surgery is the loss of tactile feedback that can result in complications from poor tissue handling, blunt dissection of dense adhesions or inappropriate tying of sutures [75]. Other causes of complications in robotic-assisted surgery are note keeping the instruments in view, defects in protective sheaths of the shears, collision of instruments, poor positioning of the patient, port and trocar placement, vaginal vault dehiscence and cuff infection, and lack of communication within the team.

Steep Trendelenburg is often required to expose the pelvic anatomy and the para-aortic area during oncologic surgery. Prolonged Trendelenburg can result in mild head contusion, subcutaneous ecchymosis, orbital pain and peri-orbital edema, corneal abrasion, visual loss, laryngeal edema, nerve injuries. Reducing operative time or reversing Trendelenburg after 4–5 h, restrictive fluid replacement, adequate padding at pressure points can prevent some of these complications [75].

Specific organ injuries during robotic-assisted surgery have a similar incidence than during laparoscopic surgery. A systematic review of the literature comparing robotic surgery to laparotomy and conventional laparoscopy for cervical cancer shows comparable risk of urologic injuries (less than 1% bladder injuries and less than 3% ureteric injuries) [76]. Urologic injuries can be prevented by thoroughly identifying the ureter and careful surgical technique avoiding excessive devascularization of the ureter and excessive use of the cautery. The use of prophylactic stents in conventional laparoscopy and laparotomy has not shown to be cost effective for the prevention of urologic injury and has not been studied in robotic-assisted gynecologic surgery [77, 78]. Bowel and vascular injuries have a low incidence and similar causes than conventional laparoscopic surgery. Some preventive measures can be used to reduce injury during entrance to the abdominal cavity but no specific technique (veress needle, open technique) has shown to be superior to prevent injuries. Good surgical technique with good exposure and correct use of electric energy are important to prevent injuries. The majority of bowel injuries are recognized intra-operatively (87%) and repaired by minimally invasive approach (58%) [79]. Nerve injuries can occur due to poor patient positioning but also during lymph node dissection (genitofemoral nerve, obturator nerve) and parametrial dissection (para-sympathetic plexus) during radical hysterectomy. Although vaginal cuff dehiscence is uncommon, it is more prevalent in robotic surgery than conventional laparoscopy, laparotomy and vaginal surgery. It is reported in up to 1.5% of hysterectomies done for benign disease and up to 2.5% for oncologic disease [80, 81]. Several measures are recommended to limit the incidence of vaginal cuff dehiscence like the use of cutting mode electrocautery during the colpotomy to reduce thermal injury, incorporating 5 mm of healthy tissue from the vaginal edge, incorporating the posterior peritoneum and uterosacral ligaments for better support and avoiding vaginal trauma (intercourse, tampons, Valsalva) for 6–12 weeks [75]. In a review of the United States Food and Drug Administration (FDA) Manufacture and User Device Experience (MAUDE) Database reporting of gynecologic robotic procedures (the majority of which consisted of robotic hysterectomy) for the year 2012, risk of major operative injury was 0.08% and the risk of death was 0.007% [82].

8. Information for patients

Patients should be provided instructions regarding perioperative information and expectations. Patients should remain NPO starting at the 12 am hour before surgery. Bowel preparation is not necessary unless bowel resection is anticipated. Prior to proceeding to the operating room patients will review and sign procedure consents with their surgeon. Detailed information regarding possible intraoperative complications is detailed above in Section 7. In general patients should be made aware that risks of robotic assisted laparoscopic hysterectomy include but not be limited to vascular injury, hemorrhage, infection, injury to bowel, bladder, ureters, nerves, and other structures adjacent to the operative field. Patients should be informed that the risk of major morbidity and death are both small (approximately <1% and <0.01% respectively) [82]. In some cases reoperation with additional surgical interventions such as bowel resection with reanastamosis and/or diversion and ureteral reimplantation may be necessary. Major causes of postoperative morbidity include sepsis and venous thromboembolism. Prophylactic antibiotics and pharmacologic anticoagulation are often administered to minimize these risks. The majority of patients undergoing robotic hysterectomy are discharged home within 24–48 h of surgery, with a large portion of patients going home on the same day as surgery.

9. Conclusion

The da Vinci Surgical System is an innovative technology that has advanced the laparoscopic treatment of benign and malignant diseases in gynecology. Da Vinci assisted laparoscopic hysterectomy has advantages over open, traditional laparoscopic, and even vaginal approaches in some cases. This surgical technique is proliferating and being adopted by university and community hospitals across the country. As the literature on the benefits of da Vinci assisted hysterectomy continues to grow, so does operator proficiency and its use in operating rooms. The newer da Vinci models have increased movement efficiency and visual capacity. Although the future utility of robotic surgeries and robotic hysterectomies necessitates further research, the potential application of this surgical method affords great promise.

Author details

Adrian Kohut[1], Leah Goldberg[1] and Alexandre Buckley De Meritens[1,2]*

*Address all correspondence to: ab1641@cinj.rutgers.edu

1 Department of Obstetrics, Gynecology, and Reproductive Sciences, Rutgers Robert Wood Johnson Medical School, Robert Wood Johnson University Hospital, New Brunswick, NJ, United States

2 Division of Gynecologic Oncology, Rutgers Cancer Institute of New Jersey, Robert Wood Johnson University Hospital, New Brunswick, NJ, United States

References

[1] Ballantyne GH, Moll F. The da Vinci telerobotic surgical system: The virtual operative field and telepresence surgery. The Surgical Clinics of North America. 2003;**83**(6):1293-1304 vii

[2] Intuitive Surgical, I. The da Vinci Surgical System. 2017. Available from: https://intuitive-surgical.com/products/davinci_surgical_system/ [cited 2017]

[3] Diaz-Arrastia C et al. Laparoscopic hysterectomy using a computer-enhanced surgical robot. Surgical Endoscopy. 2002;**16**(9):1271-1273

[4] Lambaudie E et al. Robot-assisted laparoscopy in gynecologic oncology. Surgical Endoscopy. 2008;**22**(12):2743-2747

[5] Lauterbach R, Matanes E, Lowenstein L. Review of robotic surgery in gynecology—The future is here. Rambam Maimonides Medical Journal. 2017;**8**(2):1-12

[6] Gala RB et al. Systematic review of robotic surgery in gynecology: Robotic techniques compared with laparoscopy and laparotomy. Journal of Minimally Invasive Gynecology. 2014;**21**(3):353-361

[7] Moukarzel LA, Fader AN, Tanner EJ. Feasibility of robotic-assisted laparoendoscopic single-site surgery in the gynecologic oncology setting. Journal of Minimally Invasive Gynecology. 2017;**24**(2):258-263

[8] Whiteman MK et al. Inpatient hysterectomy surveillance in the United States, 2000-2004. American Journal of Obstetrics and Gynecology. 2008;**198**(1):34e1-34e7

[9] Wright JD et al. Robotically assisted vs laparoscopic hysterectomy among women with benign gynecologic disease. JAMA. 2013;**309**(7):689-698

[10] Committee on Gynecologic, P. Committee Opinion No 701: Choosing the Route of Hysterectomy for Benign Disease. Obstetrics and Gynecology. 2017;**129**(6):e155-e159

[11] Aarts JW et al. Surgical approach to hysterectomy for benign gynaecological disease. Cochrane Database of Systematic Reviews. 2015;**8**:CD003677

[12] Ho C et al. In Robot-Assisted Surgery Compared with Open Surgery and Laparoscopic Surgery: Clinical Effectiveness and Economic Analyses. Ottawa, ON: Canadian Agency for Drugs and Technologies in Health. 2011

[13] Landeen LB et al. Clinical and cost comparisons for hysterectomy via abdominal, standard laparoscopic, vaginal and robot-assisted approaches. South Dakota Medicine. 2011;**64**(6):197-199, 201, 203 passim

[14] Geppert B, Lonnerfors C, Persson J. Robot-assisted laparoscopic hysterectomy in obese and morbidly obese women: Surgical technique and comparison with open surgery. Acta Obstetricia et Gynecologica Scandinavica. 2011;**90**(11):1210-1217

[15] Lim PC et al. Multicenter analysis comparing robotic, open, laparoscopic, and vaginal hysterectomies performed by high-volume surgeons for benign indications. International Journal of Gynaecology and Obstetrics. 2016;**133**(3):359-364

[16] Scandola M et al. Robot-assisted laparoscopic hysterectomy vs traditional laparoscopic hysterectomy: Five metaanalyses. Journal of Minimally Invasive Gynecology. 2011;**18**(6):705-715

[17] Orady M et al. Comparison of robotic-assisted hysterectomy to other minimally invasive approaches. JSLS. 2012;**16**(4):542-548

[18] Rosero EB et al. Comparison of robotic and laparoscopic hysterectomy for benign gynecologic disease. Obstetrics and Gynecology. 2013;**122**(4):778-786

[19] Surgical I. da Vinci Xi Surgical System. 2017. Available from: https://www.intuitivesurgical.com/products/da-vinci-xi/ [cited 9/29/2017]

[20] Committee opinion no. 628: Robotic surgery in gynecology. Obstetrics and Gynecology. 2015;**125**(3):760-7

[21] Sarlos D et al. Robotic hysterectomy versus conventional laparoscopic hysterectomy: Outcome and cost analyses of a matched case-control study. European Journal of Obstetrics, Gynecology, and Reproductive Biology. 2010;**150**(1):92-96

[22] Matthews CA et al. Evaluation of the introduction of robotic technology on route of hysterectomy and complications in the first year of use. American Journal of Obstetrics and Gynecology. 2010;**203**(5):499e1-499e5

[23] Payne TN, Dauterive FR. A comparison of total laparoscopic hysterectomy to robotically assisted hysterectomy: Surgical outcomes in a community practice. Journal of Minimally Invasive Gynecology. 2008;**15**(3):286-291

[24] Kilic GS et al. Comparison of perioperative outcomes of total laparoscopic and robotically assisted hysterectomy for benign pathology during introduction of a robotic program. Obstetrics and Gynecology International. 2011;**2011**:683703

[25] Shashoua AR, Gill D, Locher SR. Robotic-assisted total laparoscopic hysterectomy versus conventional total laparoscopic hysterectomy. JSLS. 2009;**13**(3):364-369

[26] Nezhat C et al. Laparoscopic hysterectomy with and without a robot: Stanford experience. JSLS. 2009;**13**(2):125-128

[27] Yamasato K et al. Effect of robotic surgery on hysterectomy trends: Implications for resident education. Journal of Minimally Invasive Gynecology. 2014;21(3):399-405

[28] Network NCC. NCCN Clinical Practice Guidelines in Oncology: Uterine Neoplasms. 2016

[29] Walker JL et al. Recurrence and survival after random assignment to laparoscopy versus laparotomy for comprehensive surgical staging of uterine cancer: Gynecologic Oncology Group LAP2 Study. Journal of Clinical Oncology. 2012;30(7):695-700

[30] Zhao Y et al. Laparoscopic radical hysterectomy in early stage cervical cancer: A systematic review and meta-analysis. Journal of Laparoendoscopic & Advanced Surgical Techniques. Part A. 2017;27(11):1132-1144

[31] Bogani G et al. Laparoscopic versus open abdominal management of cervical cancer: Long-term results from a propensity-matched analysis. Journal of Minimally Invasive Gynecology. 2014;21(5):857-862

[32] Liu Z et al. Superiority of robotic surgery for cervical cancer in comparison with traditional approaches: A systematic review and meta-analysis. International Journal of Surgery. 2017;40:145-154

[33] Gehrig PA et al. What is the optimal minimally invasive surgical procedure for endometrial cancer staging in the obese and morbidly obese woman? Gynecologic Oncology. 2008;111(1):41-45

[34] Bell MC et al. Comparison of outcomes and cost for endometrial cancer staging via traditional laparotomy, standard laparoscopy and robotic techniques. Gynecologic Oncology. 2008;111(3):407-411

[35] Lim PC, Kang E, Park DH. Learning curve and surgical outcome for robotic-assisted hysterectomy with lymphadenectomy: Case-matched controlled comparison with laparoscopy and laparotomy for treatment of endometrial cancer. Journal of Minimally Invasive Gynecology. 2010;17(6):739-748

[36] Magrina JF et al. Robotic surgery for endometrial cancer: Comparison of perioperative outcomes and recurrence with laparoscopy, vaginal/laparoscopy and laparotomy. European Journal of Gynaecological Oncology. 2011;32(5):476-480

[37] Seamon LG et al. Comprehensive surgical staging for endometrial cancer in obese patients: Comparing robotics and laparotomy. Obstetrics and Gynecology. 2009;114(1):16-21

[38] DeNardis SA et al. Robotically assisted laparoscopic hysterectomy versus total abdominal hysterectomy and lymphadenectomy for endometrial cancer. Gynecologic Oncology. 2008;111(3):412-417

[39] ElSahwi KS et al. Comparison between 155 cases of robotic vs. 150 cases of open surgical staging for endometrial cancer. Gynecologic Oncology. 2012;124(2):260-264

[40] Subramaniam A et al. A cohort study evaluating robotic versus laparotomy surgical outcomes of obese women with endometrial carcinoma. Gynecologic Oncology. 2011;122(3):604-607

[41] Barnett JC et al. Cost comparison among robotic, laparoscopic, and open hysterectomy for endometrial cancer. Obstetrics and Gynecology. 2010;**116**(3):685-693

[42] Boggess JF et al. A case-control study of robot-assisted type III radical hysterectomy with pelvic lymph node dissection compared with open radical hysterectomy. American Journal of Obstetrics and Gynecology. 2008;**199**(4):357e1-357e7

[43] Soliman PT et al. Radical hysterectomy: A comparison of surgical approaches after adoption of robotic surgery in gynecologic oncology. Gynecologic Oncology. 2011;**123**(2): 333-336

[44] Cantrell LA et al. Survival outcomes for women undergoing type III robotic radical hysterectomy for cervical cancer: A 3-year experience. Gynecologic Oncology. 2010;**117**(2): 260-265

[45] Geisler JP et al. Robotically assisted laparoscopic radical hysterectomy compared with open radical hysterectomy. International Journal of Gynecological Cancer. 2010;**20**(3): 438-442

[46] Nam EJ et al. A case-control study of robotic radical hysterectomy and pelvic lymphadenectomy using 3 robotic arms compared with abdominal radical hysterectomy in cervical cancer. International Journal of Gynecological Cancer. 2010;**20**(7):1284-1289

[47] Holloway RW et al. Comparison of total laparoscopic and abdominal radical hysterectomy for patients with early-stage cervical cancer. Obstetrics and Gynecology. 2007;**110**(5):1174, author reply 1174-5

[48] Magrina JF. Robotic surgery in gynecology. European Journal of Gynaecological Oncology. 2007;**28**(2):77-82

[49] Puntambekar SP et al. Laparoscopic total radical hysterectomy by the Pune technique: Our experience of 248 cases. Journal of Minimally Invasive Gynecology. 2007;**14**(6):682-689

[50] Obermair A et al. A phase III randomized clinical trial comparing laparoscopic or robotic radical hysterectomy with abdominal radical hysterectomy in patients with early stage cervical cancer. Journal of Minimally Invasive Gynecology. 2008;**15**(5):584-588

[51] Estape R et al. A case matched analysis of robotic radical hysterectomy with lymphadenectomy compared with laparoscopy and laparotomy. Gynecologic Oncology. 2009;**113**(3): 357-361

[52] Fanning J, Fenton B, Purohit M. Robotic radical hysterectomy. American Journal of Obstetrics and Gynecology. 2008;**198**(6):649e1-649e4

[53] Kim YT et al. Robotic radical hysterectomy with pelvic lymphadenectomy for cervical carcinoma: A pilot study. Gynecologic Oncology. 2008;**108**(2):312-316

[54] Maggioni A et al. Robotic approach for cervical cancer: Comparison with laparotomy: A case control study. Gynecologic Oncology. 2009;**115**(1):60-64

[55] Nezhat FR et al. Robotic radical hysterectomy versus total laparoscopic radical hysterectomy with pelvic lymphadenectomy for treatment of early cervical cancer. JSLS. 2008;**12**(3):227-237

[56] Persson J et al. Robot assisted laparoscopic radical hysterectomy and pelvic lymphadenectomy with short and long term morbidity data. Gynecologic Oncology. 2009;**113**(2): 185-190

[57] Sert BM, Abeler VM. Robotic-assisted laparoscopic radical hysterectomy (Piver type III) with pelvic node dissection—Case report. European Journal of Gynaecological Oncology. 2006;**27**(5):531-533

[58] Sert B, Abeler V. Robotic radical hysterectomy in early-stage cervical carcinoma patients, comparing results with total laparoscopic radical hysterectomy cases. The future is now? International Journal of Medical Robotics. 2007;**3**(3):224-228

[59] Field JB et al. Computer-enhanced robotic surgery in gynecologic oncology. Surgical Endoscopy. 2007;**21**(2):244-246

[60] Kho RM et al. Robotic hysterectomy: Technique and initial outcomes. American Journal of Obstetrics and Gynecology. 2007;**197**(1):113e1-113e4

[61] van Dam PA et al. Robotic-assisted laparoscopic cytoreductive surgery for lobular carcinoma of the breast metastatic to the ovaries. Journal of Minimally Invasive Gynecology. 2007;**14**(6):746-749

[62] Bandera CA, Magrina JF. Robotic surgery in gynecologic oncology. Current Opinion in Obstetrics & Gynecology. 2009;**21**(1):25-30

[63] Choi SB et al. Early experiences of robotic-assisted laparoscopic liver resection. Yonsei Medical Journal. 2008;**49**(4):632-638

[64] Nadeem R, Abu-Rustum RRB, Douglas A. Levine, Atlas of Procedures in Gynecologic Oncology. 3rd ed. CRC Press Taylor and Francis Group, Third Edition; 2013. p. 472

[65] Jung YW et al. The feasibility of scarless single-port transumbilical total laparoscopic hysterectomy: Initial clinical experience. Surgical Endoscopy. 2010;**24**(7):1686-1692

[66] Kim YW et al. Single-port laparoscopic myomectomy using a new single-port transumbilical morcellation system: Initial clinical study. Journal of Minimally Invasive Gynecology. 2010;**17**(5):587-592

[67] Kim TJ et al. Single port access laparoscopic adnexal surgery. Journal of Minimally Invasive Gynecology. 2009;**16**(5):612-615

[68] Ramirez PT. Single-port laparoscopic surgery: Is a single incision the next frontier in minimally invasive gynecologic surgery? Gynecologic Oncology. 2009;**114**(2):143-144

[69] Fader AN, Escobar PF. Laparoendoscopic single-site surgery (LESS) in gynecologic oncology: Technique and initial report. Gynecologic Oncology. 2009;**114**(2):157-161

[70] Paek J et al. Robotic single-site versus laparoendoscopic single-site hysterectomy: A propensity score matching study. Surgical Endoscopy. 2016;**30**(3):1043-1050

[71] Lopez S, Mulla Z, Hernandez L, Garza DM, Payne TN, Farnam RW. A comparison of outcomes between robotic-assisted, single-site laparoscopy versus laparoendoscopic single site for benign hysterectomy. Journal of Minimally Invasive Gynecology. 2016;**23**(1)

[72] Gungor M et al. Single-port hysterectomy: Robotic versus laparoscopic. Journal of Robotic Surgery. Mar 2018;**12**(1):87-92

[73] Buckley de Meritens A et al. Feasibility and learning curve of robotic laparoendoscopic single-site surgery in gynecology. Journal of Minimally Invasive Gynecology. 2017; **24**(2):323-328

[74] Manoucheri MAUDE: analysis of robotic-assisted gynecologic surgery. Journal of Minimally Invasive Gynecology. Jul-Aug 2014;**21**(4):592-595

[75] Tse KY et al. Robot-assisted gynaecological cancer surgery-complications and prevention. Best Practice and Research Clinical Obstretrics and Gynaecology. Nov 2017;**45**:94-106

[76] Park DA, Yun JE, Kim SW, et al. Surgical and clinical safety and effectiveness of robotas-sisted laparoscopic hysterectomy compared to conventional laparoscopy and laparot-omy for cervical cancer: A systematic review and meta-analysis. European Journal of Surgical Oncology. Sep 2016;**42**(9):1303-14

[77] Merritt AJ, Crosbie EJ, Charova J, et al. Prophylactic pre-operative bilateral ureteric catheters for major gynaecological surgery. Archives of Gynecology and Obstetrics. 2013;**288**:1061-1066

[78] Han L, Cao R, Jiang JY, et al. Preset ureter catheter in laparoscopic radical hysterectomy of cervical cancer. Genetics and Molecular Research. 2014;**13**:3638-3645

[79] Picerno T, Sloan NL, Escobar P, et al. Bowel injury in robotic gynecologic surgery: Risk factors and management options. A systematic review. American Journal of Obstetrics and Gynecology. 2017;**216**:10-26

[80] Landeen LB, Hultgren EM, Kapsch TM, Mallory PW. Vaginal cuff dehiscence: A random-ized trial comparing robotic vaginal cuff closure methods. Journal of Robotic Surgery. 2016;**10**(4):337-341

[81] Drudi L, Press JZ, Lau S, et al. Vaginal vault dehiscence after robotic hysterectomy for gynecologic cancers: Search for risk factors and literature review. International Journal of Gynecological Cancer. 2013;**23**:943-950

[82] Shields K, Minion L, Sumner D, Monk B. Ten year food and drug administration reporting of robot-assisted laparoscopy complications, deaths, and device malfunctions in gyneco-logic surgery. Gynecologic Oncology. 2014;**135**(2):402. DOI: 10.1016/j.ygyno.2014.07.061

9

Diagnostic Laparoscopy for Abdominal Tuberculosis: A Promising Tool for Diagnosis

Arshad M. Malik

Abstract

Introduction: Abdominal tuberculosis has plagued the mankind over several decades and is a major reason of morbidity and mortality even today in the developing world. It's a difficult problem to diagnose as most patients present with vague and nonspecific symptomatology. This study was performed with a view to find out an efficient and practical tool for diagnosing this problem.

Methods: This analytical descriptive study including 283 patients of abdominal tuberculosis is a continuation of an earlier study by the author in the same context. The study was conducted to highlight the usefulness of diagnostic laparoscopy in patients with vague abdominal symptoms, posing difficulty in establishing a conclusive diagnosis. The study extended over a nine-year period in a teaching hospital as well as some private hospitals. The data was collected and statistically analyzed on SPSS version 22.

Results: We had a total of 266 patients with unsettled diagnosis having vague abdominal symptoms. Out of the total study subjects, 214 (80.45%) were finally conclusively diagnosed to have abdominal tuberculosis on diagnostic laparoscopy. Abdominal pain is the most frequent symptom which makes the patients seek medical advice coupled with changing bowel habits, loss of weight and generalized weakness. Laparoscopy revealed various tuberculous lesions which were biopsied and diagnosed.

Conclusion: Diagnostic laparoscopy is a potential answer for the diagnostic dilemma posed by abdominal tuberculosis. Its efficacy and reliability need further studies in future.

Keywords: abdominal tuberculosis, diagnostic dilemma, morbidity, cost-effectiveness

1. Background

Abdominal tuberculosis remains one of the commonest and most difficult diseases globally as far as the diagnosis is concerned [1–5]. It is also one of the common extra-pulmonary sites for tuberculous lesions. The disease may affect any part of the gut and may produce a chronic illness with vague abdominal symptoms or else may present in an acute obstructive form. The gravity of this problem is further increased by the vague and totally non-specific symptomatology [6–7]. The presentation of abdominal tuberculosis always mimics many other conditions like inflammatory bowel diseases and other similar conditions [8–10]. This state of confusion usually leads to an undue delay in diagnosis and treatment plan and thus further increases the overall morbidity. A large number of these patients present with acute abdomen and are diagnosed on exploratory laparotomy only. This actually has been a practice in our setup where a large number of patients undergo unnecessary laparotomies. These laparotomies could be easily avoided had there been an efficient and reliable method to diagnose abdominal tuberculosis. This actually led to the consideration of diagnostic laparoscopy in all patients with suspected abdominal tuberculosis to find out tuberculous lesions and to take biopsy of any such foci. This proved to be a breakthrough with a very encouraging result [11–13]. The study focused on the possible role of laparoscopy to establish the histopathological diagnosis of tuberculosis in patients having a high degree of suspicion but we found it difficult to establish a concrete diagnosis. Early diagnosis and starting anti-tuberculous diagnosis and an early resort to the anti-tuberculous treatment can coma after morbidity can facilitate an early recovery and an early return to work. This has a lot of benefits to the patient, the community and a major cut short on the health facility.

1.2. Pathology and pathogenesis

Tuberculosis is a common problem in developing countries like Pakistan, India, Bangladesh, etc. In the early 1990s, it was considered a lethal disease as there were no medications effective against the tubercle bacillus. With the advent of anti-tuberculous drugs, the disease is no more a problem as it used to be in the past. The disease represents one of the most dreaded forms of extra-pulmonary disease and can affect virtually all parts of the GIT including intestines and various abdominal viscera.

The portal of entry of mycobacterium into the GIT is through ingestion of the infected sputum, via blood, or there may be a direct spread from infected contiguous organs like fallopian tubes, etc. [14]. The abdominal tuberculosis is divided into the following categories based on the gross appearance and involvement of the target tissue.

A. Intestinal tuberculosis

B. Glandular tuberculosis

C. Peritoneal tuberculosis

D. Solid organs

Rathi et al. [15] claim that abdominal tuberculosis constitutes 11% of the extra-pulmonary sites and the commonest area affected is the ileocecal region. The intestinal tuberculosis usually has three gross pathological forms as under

a. Hypertrophied

b. Ulcerative

c. Stricturous

The ileocecal tuberculosis is always a hypertrophied lesion which may present with acute intestinal obstruction. The ulcerative lesion is in the form of mucosal ulcers which usually present with diarrhoea and other abdominal symptoms. There is a recent claim that the extra-pulmonary manifestations of tuberculosis are observed with increasing frequency in Immuno-suppressed patients and more so with HIV patients as an accompaniment of the chronic illness [16]. An early diagnosis is the key to a curable non-operative treatment as a vast majority of these patients can be treated by anti-tuberculous drugs and thus can be saved from an undue laparotomy. In order to achieve this goal, the first and the foremost thing is to have a high index of suspicion about this entity [17] coupled with expertise in the laparoscopic technique.

2. Methods

This analytical descriptive study was conducted in a teaching hospital as well as some private hospitals. The study subjects attended the outpatient department with acute or chronic presentations. Patients having a totally confusing symptomatology and vague symptoms where a firm conclusive diagnosis could not be established were included in the study and were informed about the purpose of the study and the possible outcome. Having learnt the objectives of the study, only those who gave their consent were enrolled and admitted in the hospital. Patients who were already diagnosed as ileocecal tuberculosis or were on anti-tuberculous treatment were excluded. Upon arrival, the initial management was totally determined by the mode of presentation. Patients with acute presentation were resuscitated with I/V fluids and decompressed by nasogastric suction to stabilize for intervention. The patients who presented with vague abdominal symptoms were thoroughly examined and were given conservative treatment to correct body fluids and electrolytes and to relieve pain.

After having done the initial resuscitation and management, investigations were sent including blood complete picture, chest x-ray, abdominal x-rays, ultrasound examination and CT scan in some patients. Failing to achieve a conclusive clue on abdominal examination and investigations, a diagnostic laparoscopy was planned, keeping in view a very high incidence of the tuberculosis in our part of the world. The various variables studied included demographics, clinical presentations, common laboratory results and outcomes of diagnostic laparoscopy.

3. Results

Of the total study subjects, 266 patients were chosen for diagnostic laparoscopy based on the fact that their findings and symptomatology were so vague that a conclusion could not be drawn from the clinical examination and the usual laboratory workup. The demographics included 186 (70%) males and 80 (30%) females with a mean age of 36.59, range of 48 (17–65) and a standard deviation of 10.875. The main symptoms and the mode of presentation of the patients are shown in **Table 1**. The minimum duration of the symptoms was found to be eight days (3%), while the maximum duration of symptoms was found to be > 1 month (43%). A vast majority (81%) of the patients were found to have haemoglobin < 10 G%. Ultrasound examination was not a very helpful tool as depicted in **Table 2**. The Mantoux test was positive only in eight (3%) patients while 97% had a negative Mantoux. Erythrocyte sedimentation rate (ESR) was raised in a high number of patients (97%). Generalised tenderness of abdomen and weakness was present in 88% of the study population, while the remaining patients had insignificant examination findings. Chest x-ray was absolutely normal in 250 (94%) of the total study subjects. The various laparoscopic findings are shown in **Table 3**. One hundred and seventy-eight (67%) patients had a positive history of taking off and on anti-tuberculous medication prescribed by the local general practitioners. Most of the patients, referred from far flung areas, referred from remote far flung areas had positive laparoscopic findings compared to the urban population ($p < 0.001$). Of the total population, we were able to confirm histopathological diagnosis in 259 patients having different forms of abdominal tuberculosis. The various tuberculous findings on laparoscopy are found in **Figures 1–3**. Stricturous pathology and obstructive ileocecal tuberculosis needed operative intervention in 23 (9%) patients while remaining patients received a full course of anti-tuberculous drugs and showed full recovery. A follow-up of these patients was carried for a period of three years.

	Main symptoms			
	Sub-acute intestinal obstruction	Vague abdominal pain and loss of weight	Chronic off-and on-obstruction	Total
Mode of presentation				
Acute	0	0	12	12
Chronic	2	180	0	182
Acute-on-chronic	66	0	6	72
Total	68	180	18	266

Table 1. Mode of presentations and main symptoms.

	Frequency	Percentage	Total
Inconclusive	150	56	
Diagnosed tuberculosis	34	12.78	266
Gave suspicion of tuberculosis	82	30	

Table 2. Ultrasound abdomen results.

Finding	Frequency	Percentage
No abnormality detected	52	19
Miliary tuberculosis found	104	39
Mesenteric lymphadenopathy detected	90	34
Intestinal strictures found	20	7.5

Table 3. Various laparoscopic findings.

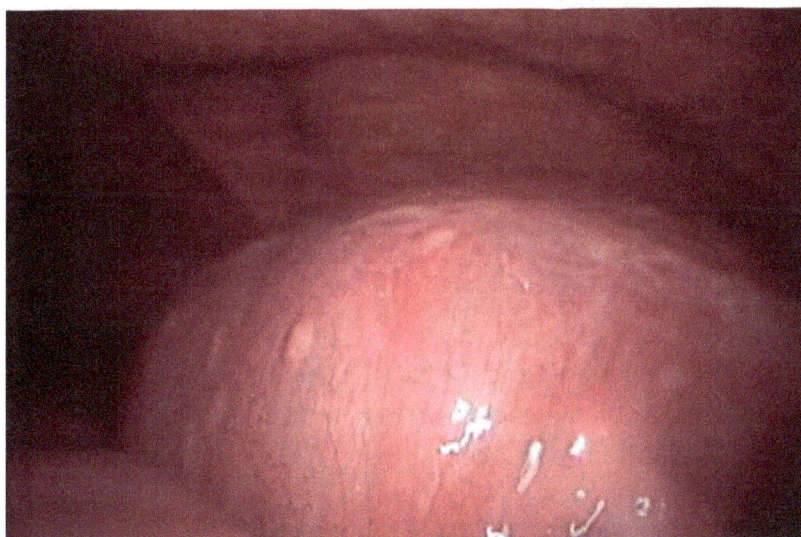

Figure 1. Miliary tubercles on the intestinal wall and abdominal wall.

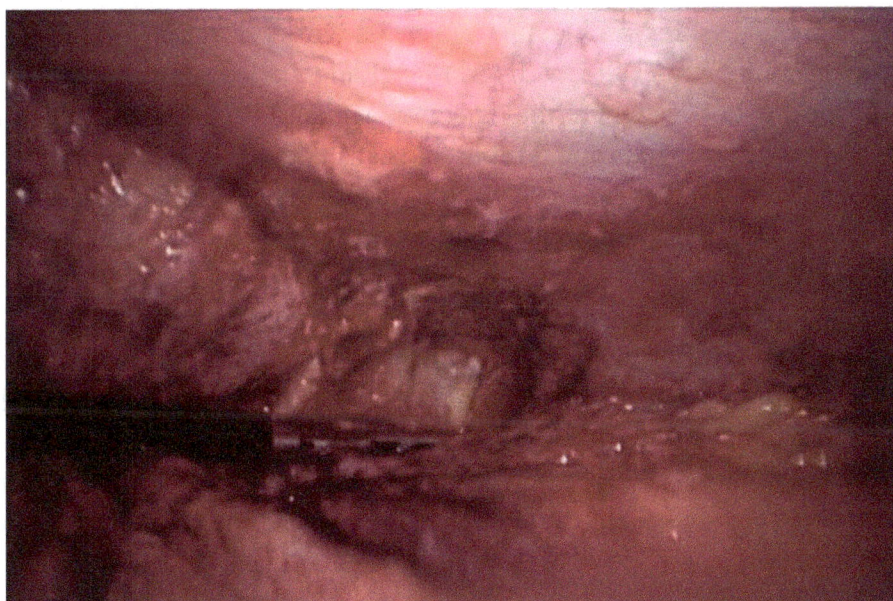

Figure 2. Plastic adhesions.

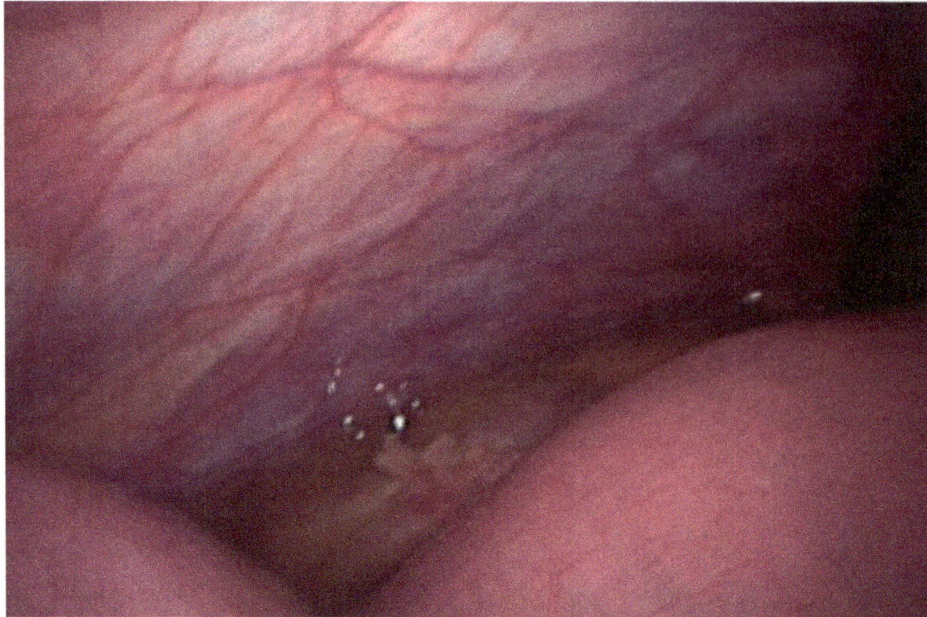

Figure 3. Ascitic fluid.

3.1. Difficulties and limitations

Although apparently an excellent diagnostic tool for the diagnosis of abdominal tuberculosis, at times we faced a lot of problems especially when there are severe plastic adhesions and more so when you find an abdominal cocoon. It is usually very difficult to introduce the first trocar in such situations.

4. Discussion

Abdominal tuberculosis remains a difficult major health issue all over the world. It is highly challenging and a dreaded problem for surgeons working in far-flung remote areas with limited resources and facilities. It is a diagnostic challenge for surgeons globally but more so in the third-world countries where the disease is rife and remains unnoticed till it turns into a serious emergency. The abdominal tuberculosis is known for its varied and confusing symptomatology whereby it mimics closely with various other similar diseases like inflammatory bowel diseases [18–19]. The unusual presentation and confusion in diagnosis usually lead to unnecessary and avoidable laparotomies, which is most of the time performed as a last resort to reach to a conclusive diagnosis. Contrary to the earlier reports, the developing countries are showing a fearful increase in the incidence of abdominal tuberculosis, as reported in recent studies [20–22]. The increase in the prevalence of abdominal tuberculosis in the developing countries is attributed to a rising incidence of HIV-positive population linking it to immunosuppression [12, 19].The age incidence of our study population coincides with other similar reports [20]. The male dominance is very clear in our studies as reported by other similar studies [18]. The varied presentation is the hallmark of abdominal tuberculosis, and as shown in our results, it is also consistent with and reported by other similar reports [23–24]. Our study highlights the fact that there is a very alarmingly high incidence of this disease in the poor, underprivileged rural population of Sind province of Pakistan. It is highly recommended to have a high level of suspicion to reach a conclusive diagnosis whenever a patient presents with vague abdominal symptoms [25]. There is hardly any absolutely reliable diagnostic test that can give a 100% confirmed diagnosis of abdominal tuberculosis. This simply is the reason for an unnecessary and life-threatening delay in the diagnosis of this disease [8, 26]. The diagnostic laparoscopy and biopsy of the tuberculous lesions are not a recent advancement but are rather known for over 30 years now [27]. It however has not been practiced widely and as commonly as it should have been. Even today, this diagnostic tool has not attracted the desired level of attention and usually is considered a last resort rather than the first in difficult diagnostic situations. In the current study, we gave it a place of primary investigation tool along with other diagnostic tests and we found it extremely encouraging as the yield of diagnosis is over 80%, in line with other similar studies [28–29]. Diagnostic laparoscopy prompts the diagnosis and can reduce the delay which can increase the morbidity and can lead to unnecessary laparotomies while improving the outcome [30–31]. Despite all the benefits, some limitations like a deceiving view leading to mis-diagnosis regardless of the experience of surgeon are mentioned by few studies [32–35].

5. Conclusion

The diagnostic laparoscopy in suspected cases of abdominal tuberculosis is an efficient and rewarding method of diagnosis. A regular use of this diagnostic modality can improve the overall outlook of this common disease in the developing world.

Author details

Arshad M. Malik

Address all correspondence to: arshadhamzapk@yahoo.com

College of Medicine, Qassim University, Saudi Arabia

References

[1] Aston NO. Abdominal tuberculosis. World J Surg 1997; 21(5):492–9.

[2] Rai S, Thomas WM. Diagnosis of abdominal tuberculosis: The importance of laparoscopy. J R Soc Med 2003; 96:586–8.

[3] Bouma BJ, Tytgat KMAJ, Shipper HG, Kager PA. Be aware of abdominal tuberculosis. Neth J Med 1997; 51:119–22.

[4]   Shakil AO, Korula J, Kanel GC, Murray NGB, Reynolds TB. Diagnostic features of tuberculous peritonitis in the absence and presence of chronic liver disease: A case control study. Am J Med 1996; 100:179–85.

[5]   Sinkala E, Gray S, Zulu I, Mudenda V, Zimba L, Vermund SH, Droniewski F, Kelly P. Clinical and ultrasonological features of abdominal tuberculosis in HIV positive adults in Zambia. BMC Infect Dis 2009; 9:44.

[6]   Uygur-Bayramicli O, Dabak G, Babak R. A clinical dilemma: Abdominal tuberculosis. World J Gastroenterol 2003; 9(5):1098–101.

[7]   Krishnan P, Vayoth SO, Dhar P et al. Laparoscopy in suspected abdominal tuberculosis is useful as an early diagnostic method. ANZ J Surg 2008; 78(11):987–9.

[8]   Akcam M, Artan R, Yilmaz A, Cig H, Aksoy NH. Abdominal tuberculosis in adolescents. Difficulties in diagnosis. Saudi Med J 2005; 26(1):122–6.

[9]   Ramesh J, Banait GS, Ormerod LP. Abdominal tuberculosis in a district general hospital: A retrospective review of 86 cases. Q J Med 2008; 101:189–95.

[10] Jaydyar H, Mindelzun RE, Olcott EW, Levitt DB. Still a great mimicker: Abdominal tuberculosis. Am J Radiol 1997; 168:1455–60.

[11] Salky BA, Edye MB. The role of laparoscopy in the diagnosis and treatment of abdominal of abdominal pain syndromes. Surg Endosc 1998; 7(12):911–4.

[12] McLaughin S, Jones T, Pitcher M, Evans P. Laparoscopic diagnosis of abdominal tuberculosis. ANZ J Surg 2008; 68(8):599–601.

[13] Sharma MP, Bhatia V. Abdominal tuberculosis. Indian J Med Res. 2004; 120(4):305–15.

[14] Rathi P, Gambhire P. Abdominal tuberculosis. J Assoc Physicians India. 2016; 64(2):38–47.

[15] Kienzl-Palma D, Prosch H. Extrathoracic manifestations of tuberculosis. Radiologe. 2016; 56(10):885–9.

[16] Debi U, Ravisankar V, Prasad KK, Sinha SK, Sharma AK. Abdominal tuberculosis of the gastrointestinal tract: Revisited. World J Gastroenterol. 2014; 20(40):14831–40. doi:10.3748/wjg.v20.i40.14831.

[17] Sinan T, Sheikh M, Ramadan S, Sahwney S, Behbehani A. CT features in abdominal tuberculosis: 20 years experience. BMC Med Imag 2002; 2(1):3.

[18] Jadvar H, Mindelzun RE, Olcott EW, Levitt DB. Still the great mimicker: Abdominal tuberculosis. Am J Roentgenol 1997; 168:1455–60.

[19] Navaneethan U, Cherian JV, Prabhu R, Venkataraman J. Distinguishing tuberculosis and Crohn's disease in developing countries: How certain can you be of the diagnosis? Saudi J Gastroenterol 2009; 15(2):142–4.

[20] Kapoor V. Abdominal tuberculosis. Medicine 2009; 35(5):257–60.

[21] Kishore PV, Palaian S, chandersekhar TS. Diagnosing tuberculosis. A retrospective study from Nepal. Internet J Gastroenterol 2008; 6(2):1–6

[22] Al Karawi MA, Mohammed AE, Yasawy MI, Graham DY, Shariq S, Ahmed AM et al. Protean manifestations of gastrointestinal tuberculosis; report on 130 patients. J Clin Gastroenterol 1995; 20(3):225–32.

[23] Tan KK, Chen K, Sim R. The spectrum of abdominal tuberculosis in a developed country: A single institutions experience over 7 years. J Gatroentrointest Surg 2009; 13(1):142–7.

[24] Vyravanathan S, Jeyarajah R. Tuberculous peritonitis: A review of thirty-five cases. Post Grad Med J 1980; 56(659):649–51.

[25] Uzunkoy A, Harma M, Harma M. Diagnosis of abdominal tuberculosis: Experience from 11 cases and review of the literature. World J Gasteroenterol 2004; 10(24):3647–9.

[26] Al Muneef M, Memish Z, Al Mahmoud S, Al Sadoon S, Bannatyne R, Khan Y. Tuberculosis in the belly: A review of forty six cases involving the gastrointestinal tract and peritoneum. Scand J Gastroenterol 2001; 36(5):528–32.

[27] Tarcoveanu E, Flip V, Moldovanu R, Dimofte G, Lupascu C, Vlad N et al. Abdominal tuberculosis- a surgical reality. Chirurgia (Bucur) 2007; 102(3):303–8.

[28] Machado N, Grant CS, Scrimgeour E. Abdominal tuberculosis—experience of a university hospital in Oman. Acta Trop 2001; 80(2):187–90.

[29] Trujillo NP. Peritoneoscopy and guided biopsy in the diagnosis of intra abdominal diseases. Gastroentrology 1976; 71:1083–5.

[30] Singh-Ranger D. Diagnosis of abdominal tuberculosis. J R Soc Med 2004; 97:154–7.

[31] Udwadia TE. Diagnostic laparoscopy. Surg Endosc 2004; 18(1):6–10.

[32] Al-Akeely MH. Impact of elective diagnostic laparoscopy in chronic abdominal disorders. Saudi J Gastroentrol 2006; 12(1):27–30.

[33] Cached J, Mekki M, Mansour A, Ben Brahim M, Maazoun K, Hidouri S et al. Contribution of laparoscopy in abdominal tuberculosis diagnosis: Retrospective study of about 11 cases. Pediatr Surg Int 2010; 26(4):413–8.

[34] Tarcoveanu E, Dimofte G, Bradea C, Lupascu C, Moldovanu R, Vasilescu A. Peritoneal tuberculosis in laparoscopic era. Acta Chir Belg 2009; 109(1):65–70.

[35] Meshikhes AW. Pitfalls of diagnostic laparoscopy in abdominal tuberculosis. Surg Endosc 2010; 24(4):908–10.

10

Autotracking Camera for Dry Box Laparoscopic Training

Masakazu Sato, Minako Koizumi, Kei Inaba,
Yu Takahashi, Natsuki Nagashima, Hiroshi Ki,
Nao Itaoka, Chiharu Ueshima, Maki Nakata and
Yoko Hasumi

Abstract

While laparoscopic surgery is less invasive than open surgery and is now common in various medical fields, laparoscopic surgery often requires more time for the operator to achieve mastery. Dry box training is one of the most important methods for developing laparoscopic skill. However, the camera is usually fixed to a particular point, which is different from practical surgery, during which the operational field is constantly adjusted by an assistant. Therefore, we introduced a camera for dry box training that can be moved by surgeons as desired by using computer vision. By detecting the ArUco marker, the camera attached onto the servomotor successfully tracked the forceps automatically. This system could easily be modified and become operable by a foot switch or voice, and collaborations between surgeons and medical engineers are expected.

Keywords: computer simulation, endoscopic surgery, robotic surgical procedures, computer vision, augmented reality

1. Introduction

Laparoscopic surgery is one of the surgical approaches, and the proportion is increasingly compared to conventional open surgery [1]. In laparoscopic surgery, surgeons use a few and small incisions (5–10 mm in general) to enter into the abdomen. Through the incision, surgeons insert specialized instruments and camera and perform surgery inside the abdomen.

While laparoscopic surgery is less invasive than conventional open surgery and is now common in various medical fields, laparoscopic surgery often requires more time for the operator to achieve mastery [2]. This is because the field of laparoscopic surgery is two-dimensional through a camera, and it takes a lot of time for surgeons who have often performed conventional open surgery to get accustomed to the camera view [2]. Thus, surgeons must practice extensively before performing practical laparoscopic surgery. Dry box training is one of the most important methods for developing laparoscopic skill [3, 4]. Dry box training consists of real instruments (such as forceps, scissors, needles, etc.) inserted into a box with a camera [5]. In general, organ models made from rubber or silicon are placed inside the box, and the surgeons practice how to use forceps, suturing, and other basic skills for laparoscopic surgery. The advantage of dry box training is the low cost. On the other hand, the camera is usually fixed to a particular point, which is different from practical surgery, during which the operational field is constantly adjusted by an assistant [5, 6]. Thus, surgeons need to manually change the camera angle to focus on where they are manipulating during training. This requirement leads to inefficiency because surgeons must pause the procedure every time they move the camera. Additionally, this inefficiency may prevent surgeons from practicing with the dry box training because some are annoyed by the interruptions. Some researchers elegantly investigated controlling camera by computer vision, but it would be expensive to introduce and not be suitable for the dry box training [7].

Therefore, we introduced a reasonable camera for dry box training that can be moved by surgeons as desired by using computer vision. In recent years, deep learning has been widely used for visual tracking in the field of computer vision analysis [8]. On the other hand, operation is now exclusively performed by single surgeon, which is called solo surgery [9]. Thus, the system which enables surgeons to be free from manipulating various instruments and to focus on surgical maneuvering will be more and more expected. In that context, artificial intelligence or deep learning has a great possibility to realize it.

This chapter is organized as follows. In Section 2, we introduce our applied methodology of autotracking camera. Section 3 deals with the results we obtained from the instrument. Section 4 covers the possibilities of computer vision in the field of surgery.

2. Methods and materials

2.1. ArUco marker

We used the OpenCV2 library for ArUco marker detection (https://opencv.org) [10, 11]. Briefly, OpenCV (Open Source Computer Vision Library) was designed for computational efficiency with a strong focus on real-time applications. Providers say that "An ArUco marker is a synthetic square marker composed by a wide black border and an inner binary matrix which determines its identifier (id). The black border facilitates its fast detection in the image and the binary codification allows its identification and the application of error detection and correction techniques. The marker size determines the size of the internal matrix. For instance, a marker size of 4 × 4 is composed by 16 bits" (https://docs.opencv.org/3.1.0/d5/dae/tutorial_aruco_detection.html). We referred to the code in the official tutorial. We printed an

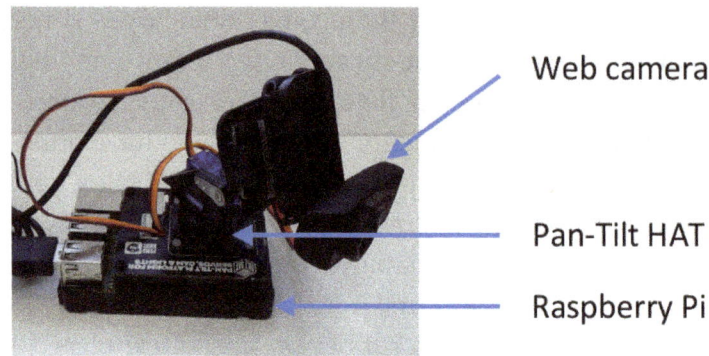

Figure 1. Raspberry Pi and Pan-Tilt HAT. A small computer, Raspberry Pi, and a servomotor, Pan-Tilt HAT, were connected, and the ordinal web camera was attached on top.

ArUco marker and attached it to the needle holder. We used the ArUco marker because of its robustness. As we recently demonstrated, the marker can be detected at a size as small as the forceps [12]. This means that their applications in the dry box training may be extended to clinical practice.

2.2. Servomotor

A servomotor is required to move the camera. In this study, we used the Pan-Tilt HAT (Pimoroni, Sheffield, United Kingdom) as the servomotor, as shown in **Figure 1** (https://shop. pimoroni.com/products/pan-tilt-hat). We rotated the servomotor to the degree at which the ArUco marker was detected. The brief rationale is as follows: first, Raspberry Pi (a small computer) obtained consecutive images through the camera and then calculated the distance from the center of the current frame image to the center of the ArUco marker when it was recognized. The distance was expressed similar to a vector: x-axis (horizontal pixel) or y-axis (vertical pixel). Then, the angles were calculated, and the servomotor was rotated according to those calculations (x-axis for a pan rotation and y-axis for a tilt rotation) [13].

We referred to the code of FaceTracker in the official tutorial (https://github.com/pimoroni/ PanTiltFacetracker). Our modified code is shown in SI Text 1.

2.3. Development environment

The development platform used in this study was Raspberry Pi 3, model B (https://www. raspberrypi.org) [12]. Raspberry Pi and Pan-Tilt HAT are shown in **Figure 1**.

3. Results

3.1. ArUco marker detection and autotracking

This investigation consists of two parts as described in Section 2. The first objective was to detect the ArUco marker, and the other objective was to track the marker by using the servomotor. As shown in **Figure 2** and Video 1, we succeeded in detecting and tracking the marker.

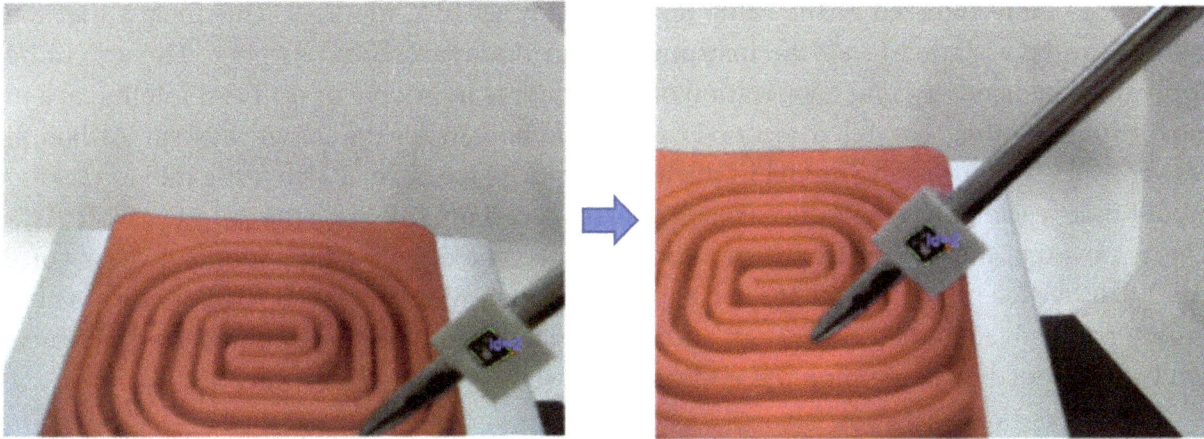

Figure 2. Autotracking model. The detected ArUco marker was automatically tracked by using the servomotor.

The ArUco marker sometimes failed to be detected, but this occurred when the marker was too far from the camera. In addition, we thought that it was not problematic as long as surgeons used the forceps for training, as the marker would typically be within the detectable range.

As shown in Video 1, the speed and smoothness of the rotation from the Pan-Tilt HAT were satisfactory. Interestingly, we felt that the Pan-Tilt HAT might be better at performing a pan rotation than a tilt rotation. This might be due to using a non-expensive machine; however, we still consider our system to be suitable for dry box training because of its low cost and simplicity to create.

4. Discussion

Herein, we introduced a camera that can be moved by surgeons as they wish. The idea of cooperative human-machine coexistence has been the most researcher's focus [14]. And, in that context, we are now interested in investigating cooperative system for surgery.

While dry box training is important for laparoscopy training, it differs from practical surgery in that the camera is usually fixed and does not move [3, 4]. Thus, surgeons need to manu-ally change the camera angle every time they would like to focus on where they are suturing, thus producing unwanted inefficiency in training. Therefore, we introduced a camera that can automatically track the forceps to which an ArUco marker has been attached.

We propose two future directions. One research direction is the method for marker detection. We detected the ArUco marker in this study; however, this marker may not always be neces-sary if the energy device or forceps can be detected by using computer vision [6]. Indeed, recent studies have investigated using an autotracking camera to track the device [15–18]. We consider these studies to be very important and may be essential for future robotic surgery. The advantage of using the ArUco marker is its robustness. As we previously described, we succeeded in detecting the ArUco marker at a size as small as the forceps [12]. Thus, we imag-ine that the marker may be used by embedding or depicting it directly on the forceps. Another advantage of using the ArUco marker is that we can use various markers at a time. The ArUco marker can be recognized at the same time as many as 1024 markers. This means that the marker can be assigned to all the instruments during laparoscopic surgery. This might be applied to the handling and cooperation of instruments by robots or artificial intelligence in the future. The other research direction is where and how to use the camera system. Although we showed an autotracking model in the present study, we have also investigated a tracking model that reacts only when the surgeon presses a certain key (e.g., the "s" key; SI Text 2). This means that the system can be modified and become operable by a foot switch or voice [19, 20]. Indeed, a robotic arm that can be operated and moved by a foot switch or voice is now commercially available [19, 21–23]. In addition, we believe that more sophisticated products can be developed by combining these ideas and systems.

5. Conclusions

We introduced a camera that can be moved by surgeons as they wish. We conclude that this investigation could easily be applied to a practical camera and robotic arm. In addition, collaborations between surgeons and medical engineers are expected.

Acknowledgements

This chapter has not been published elsewhere and is not being considered for publication in other journals.

Conflicts of interest

Authors declare that there are no conflicts of interest.

Supporting information

SI Text 1. ArUco marker tracker.

The code consists of two parts. The first part was used to detect the ArUco marker, and the other part was used to track the marker by using the servomotor.

SI Text 2 Modified ArUco marker tracker.

The model shown in SI was modified so that the camera reacted only when the surgeon pressed a certain key (e.g., the "s" key).

Video 1. ArUco marker detection and autotracking (https://www.youtube.com/watch?v= PIZod4SALsY%27%27).

The detected ArUco marker was automatically tracked by using the servomotor.

Author details

Masakazu Sato[1,2]*, Minako Koizumi[1], Kei Inaba[1], Yu Takahashi[1], Natsuki Nagashima[1], Hiroshi Ki[1], Nao Itaoka[1], Chiharu Ueshima[1], Maki Nakata[1] and Yoko Hasumi[1]

*Address all correspondence to: masakasatou-tky@umin.ac.jp

1 Department of Obstetrics and Gynecology, Mitsui Memorial Hospital, Tokyo, Japan

2 Department of Obstetrics and Gynecology, Graduate School of Medicine,
The University of Tokyo, Tokyo, Japan

References

[1] Moawad G, Liu E, Song C, Fu AZ. Movement to outpatient hysterectomy for benign indications in the United States, 2008-2014. PLoS One. 2017;**12**(11):e0188812

[2] Jaffe TA, Hasday SJ, Knol M, Pradarelli J, Quamme SRP, Greenberg CC, et al. Safety considerations in learning new procedures: a survey of surgeons. The Journal of Surgical Research. 2017;**218**:361-366

[3] Chandrasekera SK, Donohue JF, Orley D, Barber NJ, Shah N, Bishai PM, et al. Basic laparoscopic surgical training: examination of a low-cost alternative. European Urology. 2006;**50**(6):1285-1290 90-1

[4] Hinata N, Iwamoto H, Morizane S, Hikita K, Yao A, Muraoka K, et al. Dry box training with three-dimensional vision for the assistant surgeon in robot-assisted urological surgery. International Journal of Urology: Official Journal of the Japanese Urological Association. 2013;**20**(10):1037-1041

[5] Torricelli FC, Barbosa JA, Marchini GS. Impact of laparoscopic surgery training laboratory on surgeon's performance. World Journal of Gastrointestinal Surgery. 2016;**8**(11):735-743

[6] Huri E, Ezer M, Chan E. The novel laparoscopic training 3D model in urology with surgical anatomic remarks: Fresh-frozen cadaveric tissue. Turkish Journal of Urology. 2016;**42**(4):224-229

[7] Wijsman PJM, Broeders I, Brenkman HJ, Szold A, Forgione A, Schreuder HWR, et al. First experience with the autolap system: an image-based robotic camera steering device. Surgical Endoscopy. 2017

[8] Feng X, Mei W, Hu D. A review of visual tracking with deep learning. In: 2nd International Conference on Artificial Intelligence and Industrial Engineering (AIIE2016); 2016

[9] Yang YS, Kim SH, Jin CH, Oh KY, Hur MH, Kim SY, Yim HS. Solo surgeon single-port laparoscopic surgery with a homemade laparoscope-anchored instrument system in benign gynecologic diseases. Journal of Minimally Invasive Gynecology. 2014;**21**(4):695-701

[10] Shao P, Ding H, Wang J, Liu P, Ling Q, Chen J, et al. Designing a wearable navigation system for image-guided cancer resection surgery. Annals of Biomedical Engineering. 2014;**42**(11):2228-2237

[11] Zemirline A, Agnus V, Soler L, Mathoulin CL, Obdeijn M, Liverneaux PA. Augmented reality-based navigation system for wrist arthroscopy: Feasibility. Journal of Wrist Surgery. 2013;**2**(4):294-298

[12] Sato M, Koizumi M, Hino T, Takahashi Y, Nagashima N, Itaoka N, et al. Exploration of assistive technology for uniform laparoscopic surgery. Asian Journal of Endoscopic Surgery. 2018

[13] Wei CC, Song YC, Chang CC, Lin CB. Design of a solar tracking system using the brightest region in the sky image sensor. Sensors (Basel, Switzerland). 2016;**16**(12)

[14] Hamid OH, Smith NL, Barzanji A. Automation, per se, is not job elimination: How artificial intelligence forwards cooperative human-machine coexistence. In: 2017 15th International Conference on Industrial Informatics (INDIN); Germany: EmdenLeer; 2017. pp. 899-904

[15] Navarro AA, Hernansanz A, Villarraga EA, Giralt X, Aranda J. Enhancing perception in minimally invasive robotic surgery through self-calibration of surgical instruments. In: Conference Proceedings: Annual International Conference of the IEEE Engineering in Medicine and Biology Society IEEE Engineering in Medicine and Biology Society Annual Conference; 2007; 2007. pp. 457-60

[16] Toti G, Garbey M, Sherman V, Bass BL, Dunkin BJ. A smart trocar for automatic tool recognition in laparoscopic surgery. Surgical Innovation. 2015;**22**(1):77-82

[17] Voros S, Long JA, Cinquin P. Automatic localization of laparoscopic instruments for the visual servoing of an endoscopic camera holder. In: Medical Image Computing and Computer-Assisted Intervention: MICCAI International Conference on Medical Image Computing and Computer-Assisted Intervention; 2006. 9(Pt 1):pp. 535-42

[18] Zhao Z. Real-time 3D visual tracking of laparoscopic instruments for robotized endoscope holder. Bio-Medical Materials and Engineering. 2014;**24**(6):2665-2672

[19] Mewes A, Hensen B, Wacker F, Hansen C. Touchless interaction with software in interventional radiology and surgery: A systematic literature review. International Journal of Computer Assisted Radiology and Surgery. 2017;**12**(2):291-305

[20] Petroni G, Niccolini M, Caccavaro S, Quaglia C, Menciassi A, Schostek S, et al. A novel robotic system for single-port laparoscopic surgery: Preliminary experience. Surgical Endoscopy. 2013;**27**(6):1932-1937

[21] Dikici S, Aldemir Dikici B, Eser H, Gezgin E, Baser O, Sahin S, et al. Development of a 2-dof uterine manipulator with LED illumination system as a new transvaginal uterus amputation device for gynecological surgeries. Minimally Invasive Therapy & Allied

Technologies: MITAT: Official Journal of the Society for Minimally Invasive Therapy. 2017:1-9

[22] Gutierrez MM, Pedroso JD, Volker KW, Howard DL, McCarus SD. The McCarus-Volker ForniSee(R): A novel trans-illuminating colpotomy device and uterine manipulator for use in conventional and robotic-assisted laparoscopic hysterectomy. Surgical Technology International. 2017;**30**:191-196

[23] Maheshwari M, Ind T. Concurrent use of a robotic uterine manipulator and a robotic laparoscope holder to achieve assistant-less solo laparoscopy: The double ViKY. Journal of Robotic Surgery. 2015;**9**(3):211-213

11

Diastasis Recti and Other Midline Defects: Totally Subcutaneous Endoscopic Approach

Pablo José Medina, Guido Luis Busnelli and
Walter Sebastián Nardi

Abstract

Diastasis of the rectus is defined as the separation of the midline or alba line, which originates in a laxity of the interlocking fibers from the aponeurosis of both rectus muscles. At present, its surgical correction continues to be discussed. However, there is a multiplicity of factors that justify it.

Keywords: diastasis recti, endoscopic rectus plication, mini-invasive, midline defects

1. Introduction

Diastasis recti is an anatomic term used to describe a condition in which both rectus muscles are separated by a distance greater than expected. Usually caused by the reduction of the consistency of the intercrossed fibers that make the linea alba, generating a separation of both aponeurosis of the rectus abdominis muscles. It can be congenital or acquired, favored by situations like pregnancy, obesity or previous surgeries.

Clinically represents an aesthetic and symptomatic problem. It produces malfunction of the abdominal wall muscles with an associated muscular imbalance and chronic back pain [1, 2].

Nowadays, there is no consensus on the surgical technique or indications for the treatment of diastasis recti, specially in patients without lipodystrophy. If is symptomatic, causes esthetic problems (specially in young women after pregnancy [3]) or associated with midline hernias (**Figure 1a–c**), the surgical treatment of both pathologies at the same time could be recommended. The most common technique used is by the way of an abdominoplasty

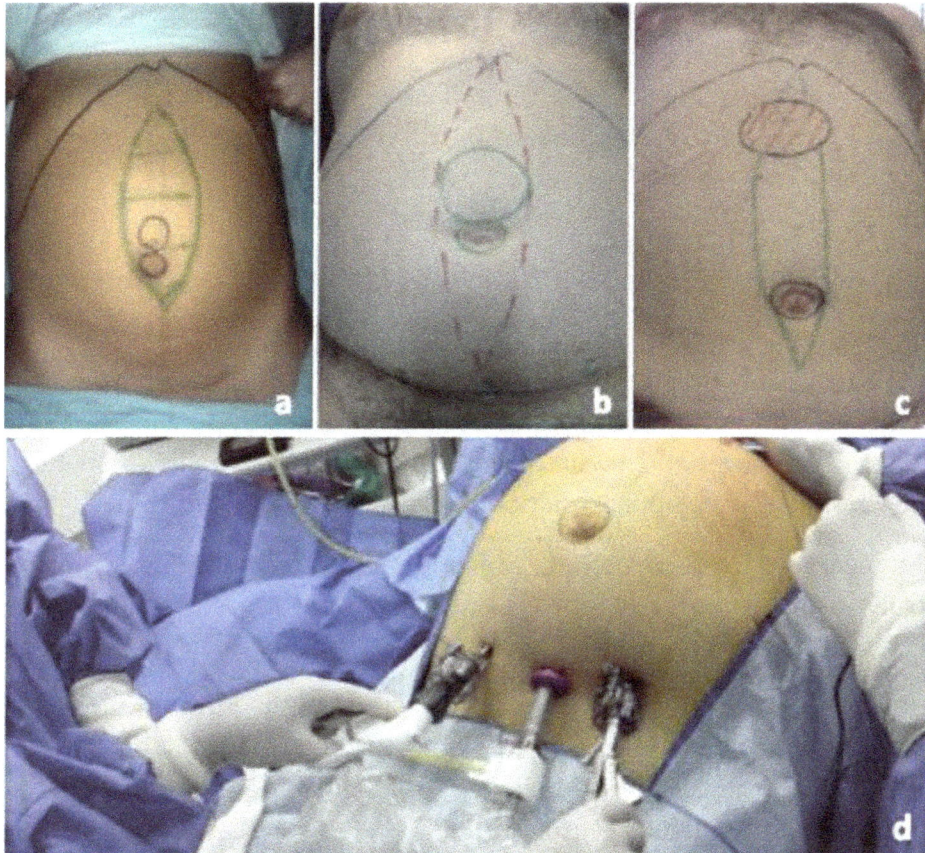

Figure 1. (a–c) External marking of the diastase recti and it's associated midline defects. (d) Position of the trocars and surgeon.

in patients with excess abdominal skin and subcutaneous cellular tissue [4]. However, a mini-invasive approach presents as an alternative procedure to the most commonly used technique for its treatment.

2. Surgical technique/technical aspects

Different options have been proposed such as conventional surgery, with abdominoplasty, laparoscopic or endoscopic approach.

For the endoscopic approach, under general anesthesia, the patient is positioned in supine position with both legs open and the surgeon is located between them. The monitor is located at the head of the patient and the assistant on his left. A 10 mm incision is made in the suprapubic midline and a space is created between the subcutaneous cellular tissue and the superficial aponeurosis with blunt dissection. A 10 mm trocar is introduced for the optic and, favored by a 10 mm Hg pneumatic pressure, two 5-mm trocars are placed under direct vision on each side of the midline by around 5 cm (**Figure 1d**).

10 mm Hg CO_2 is used to maintain a correct work space. Under endoscopic vision, the supra-aponeurotic space is dissected exposing the linea alba and superficial aponeurosis until

reaching the umbilical region. The umbilicus is disinserted above the hernia sac if present, reintroducing it into the intra-abdominal compartment. If other supraumbilical abdominal wall defects are present, the dissection is done as previously described. Finally, the dissection of the supra-aponeurotic space continues until reaching the subxiphoid region. Once dissection is completed, the diastasis recti and associated aponeurotic defects can be identified (**Figure 2a** and **b**).

The plication of the aponeurosis of the recti muscles is done with two continuous absorbable barbed sutures from the subxiphoid to suprapubic region (**Figure 2c** and **d**).

In patients with associated large abdominal wall defects, the plication of both muscles can be difficult and the release of one or both rectus abdominis muscle aponeurosis could be convenient for a tension-free plication. The *component separation technique* allows a better compliance and 4–5 cm (each side) for the approximation of the muscles to the midline.

If the defect/s measures more than 4 cm, a prosthetic material is preferred to complete the abdominal wall repair. Usually, a polypropylene mesh is introduced in the supra-aponeurotic space (onlay) and fixed with knots of an absorbable suture or tracks (**Figure 3a–c**).

Finally, the umbilicus is reinserted to its normal position to the plicated fascia with an intracorporeal knotting (**Figure 3d**). Drainage is placed through one of the 5 mm wounds used in the surgery and a compressive bandage is used to decrease the dead space between the aponeurosis and the subcutaneous cellular tissue.

For the laparoscopic approach, the patient is placed supine with both arms outstretched. The monitor is located on the right flank. Pneumoperitoneum to 12 mm Hg is achieved via open

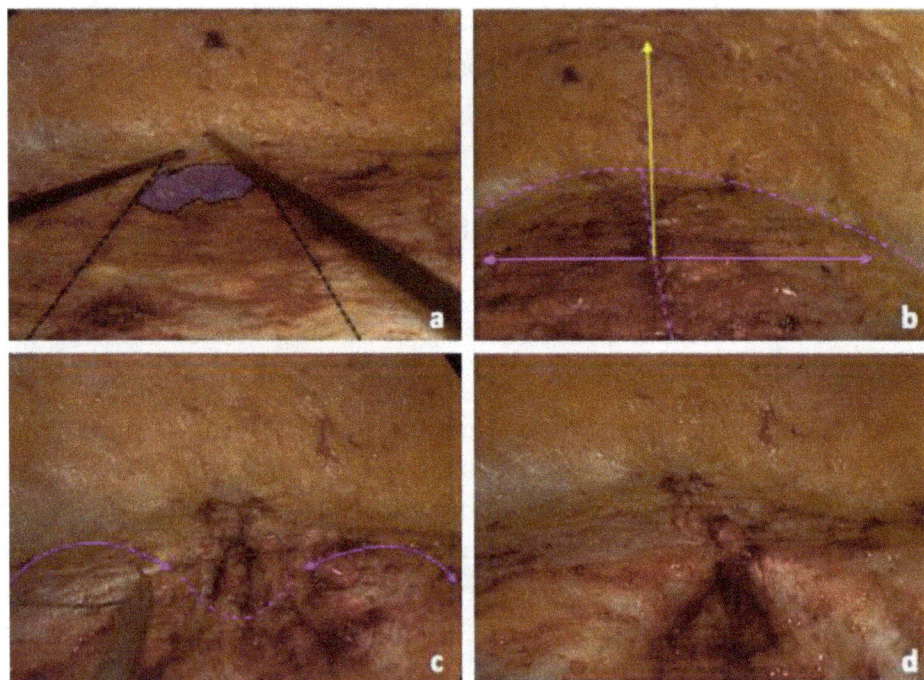

Figure 2. (a) Visualization of the diastasis recti and associated midline defect. (b) Final dissection of the supra-aponeurotic space until the subxifoid region. (c and d) Plication of the aponeurosis of diastase recti with absorbable barbed suture.

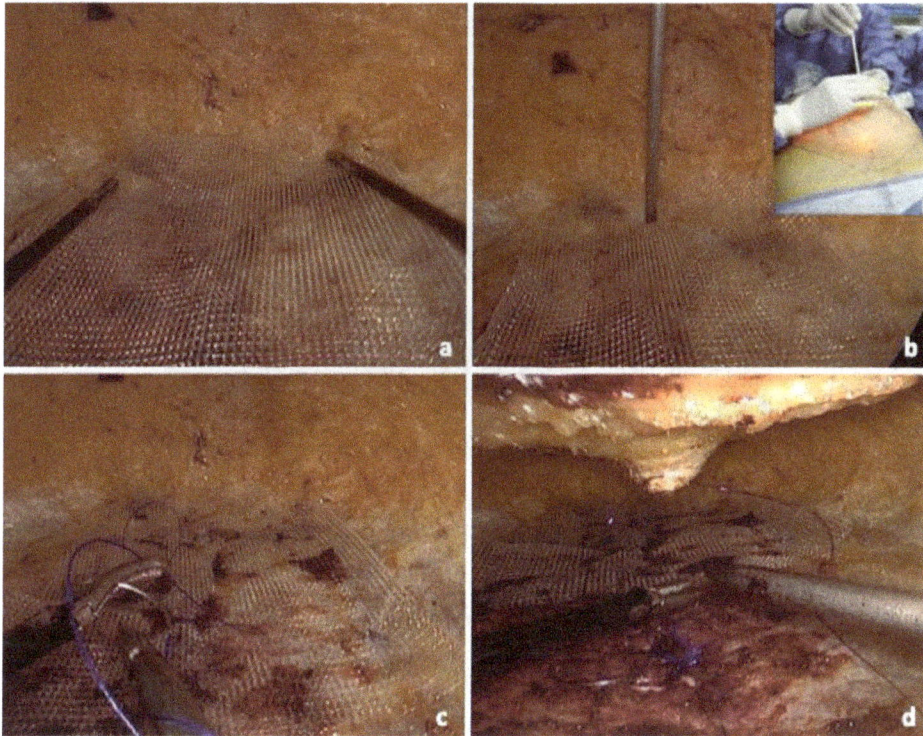

Figure 3. (a) Supra-aponeurotic polypropylene mesh is necessary to complete the abdominal wall repair. (b and c) Fixation with tracks and absorbable suture. (d) Reinsertion of the umbilicus with an intracorporeal knotting.

access of 12 mm in left flank and two additional trocars are placed in left upper quadrant (12 mm) and the left iliac fossa (5 mm).

Is better to start with laparoscopic time because sometimes is necessary to make extensive enterolysis and this is usually the most laborious process (**Figure 4**). All previous wall adhesions must be released.

Diastasis of rectus abdominis is observed and measured in all its extension (**Figure 5**).

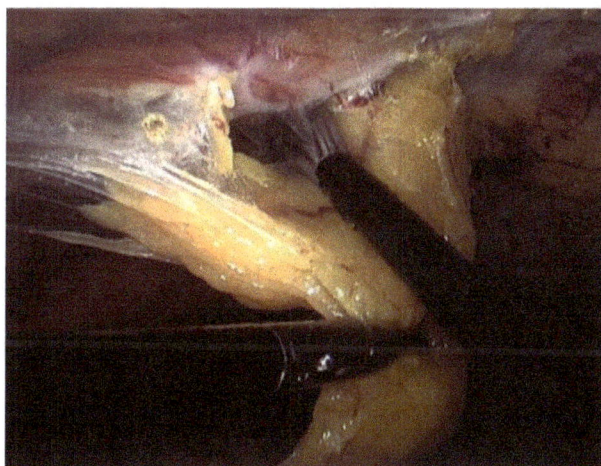

Figure 4. Release of anterior wall adhesions.

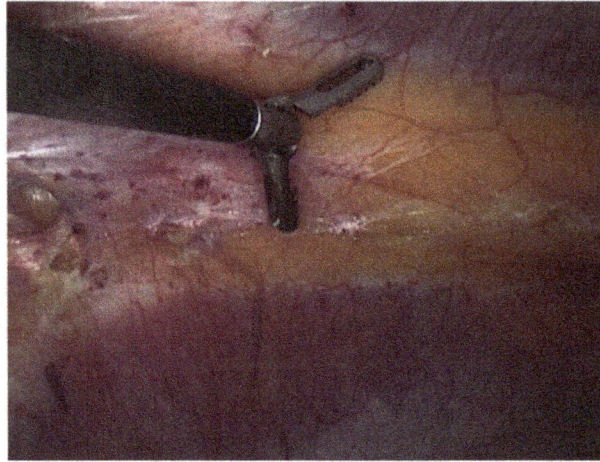

Figure 5. Measurement of diastasis recti using the diameter of the grasper.

Later on, some cases can use the *videoscopic component separation technique* to release rectus abdominis muscle and allow a tension-free plication. Exsufflation is performed and the same port sites are used. The external oblique muscle aponeurosis is identified in the upper 12 mm incision and is sectioned to access the avascular space between the external oblique and internal oblique muscles. This plane is developed with a blunt instrument. The space is then insufflated under vision and the semilunar line is visualized. The insufflation pressure is maintained at 12 mm Hg and the other two abdominal trocars are removed up to the space between both oblique muscles. This space is developed with blunt grasper maneuvers all the way between the costal margin and the inguinal ligament inferiorly. Finally, the release of the rectus is obtained by making an incision in the external oblique fascia lateral to the semilunar line. Hence, a release of the abdominis rectus sheath of about 6–8 cm is reached (**Figure 6a** and **b**). Is important to remember that nerve supply to the rectus muscle is medial to the semilunar line, hence the procedure prevents any injury to the nerves. If the diastasis is very large, greater than about 6 or 7 cm, the same procedure can be reproduced on the other side. Hemostasis is ensured and no drains are left in the dissected space. The abdominal cavity is then entered again.

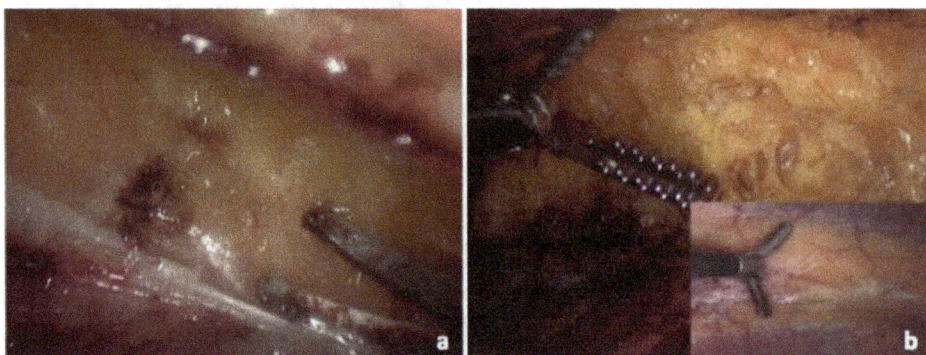

Figure 6. (a) Section of the external oblique aponeurosis. (b) Comparison between the distance between the external oblique fascia sectioned and the diameter of the diastasis.

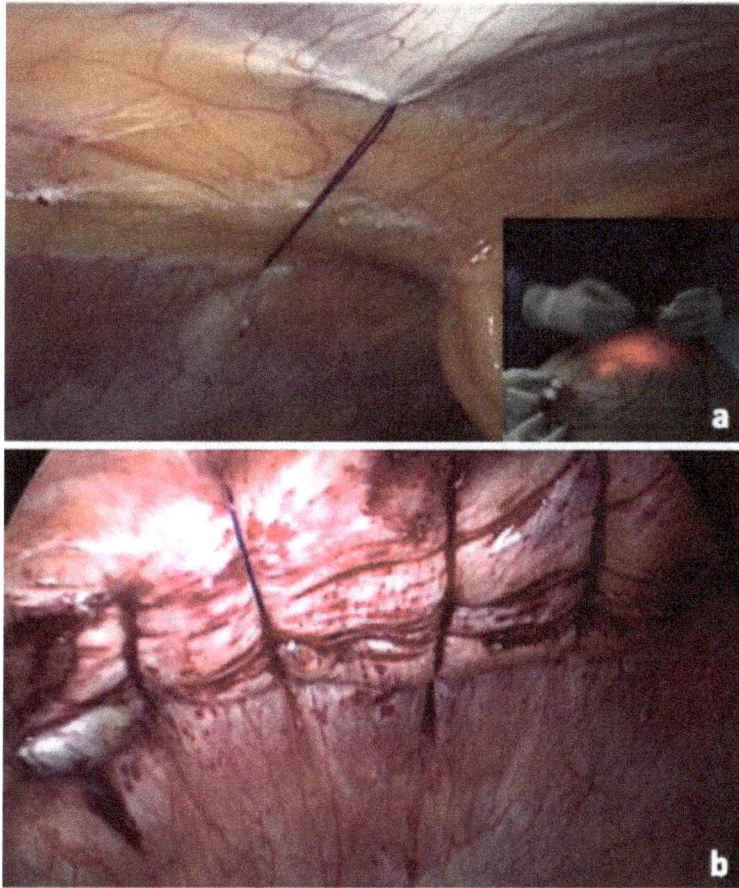

Figure 7. (a) and (b) Transmural stitches of polypropylene are placed along the entire diastasis including both rectus abdominis muscles with a laparoscopic suture passer device.

Transmural stitches of polypropylene suture are placed along the entire diastasis including both rectus abdominis muscles with a laparoscopic suture passer device such as "Endo Close™" (**Figure 7a** and **b**). Each stitch is introduced through a punctate stab incision in the skin and the knots are hidden in the subcutaneous tissue. After that, a composite mesh is prepared with permanent sutures that are placed at the midpoint of each side of the mesh before it is introduced into the abdominal cavity through a 12-mm trocar. Once the mesh is placed inside the abdominal cavity, it is secured to the abdominal wall with the preplaced sutures. Metal or absorbable tacks are then used circumferentially at approximately 1-cm intervals to prevent intestinal herniation.

3. Discussion

For the study of diastasis recti, CT scan or ultrasonography can be used. Both methods are reliable for the measurement of the separation of the rectus muscles. CT scan has the advantage of using bony ridges for that measurement and also can show other associated hernias [5]. Some authors propose that ultrasonography is an accurate method to measure rectus diastasis above the umbilicus and at the umbilical level. However, below umbilicus ultrasound can show smaller values [6].

Several ways to define and assess rectus muscle diastasis can be found in the literature. In addition, there is no consensus on the values considered relevant. Some authors consider any separation of the rectus abdominis as a diastasis and others consider a distance greater than 1 cm, 2 fingers or 3 cm.

The standard treatment of this condition is abdominoplasty with periumbilical incision, which often results in an umbilical circumcision or even an inverted T scar [7]. Limited incision abdominoplasty, sometimes called extended miniabdominoplasty, has been described in the literature but has received little attention. In conclusion, the majority of these techniques are for an open approach, while laparoscopy or endoscopy was not frequently reported at first. Nowadays plication of the diastasis without skin resection using only laparoscopic or endoscopic approach has been reported.

It is frequent to observe the coexistence of diastasis recti with one or more hernia or symptomatic incisional midline hernia. If only the hernia were treated, it would be done over an anatomic weak and deficient tissue, which is the damaged linea alba. This situation could lead to a higher possibility of hernia recurrence and also the aesthetic results would be uncertain. Thus, in these cases, simultaneous correction of all existent pathologies is highly recommended [8].

One option described for the plication of diastasis recti with skin resection is the laparoscopic approach [9]. Transmural stitches or even intracorporeal continuous suture can be done to reduce the diastasis. Finally an intra-peritoneal mesh is used to complete the procedure.

Bellido Luque et al. described the subcutaneous endoscopic approach as a new alternative to treat diastasis recti [4]. As explained before, with three supra-pubic trocars and using a pressure of CO_2 maintained between 8 and 10 mm Hg, a totally endoscopic treatment is used for the plicature of diastasis recti and also to treat associated abdominal wall defects. The utilization of barbed sutures for the plicature allows more rapid surgical maneuvers and therefore diminishing surgical times. Even though this suture is absorbable (180 days), a second continuous non-absorbable monofilament suture is added to ensure more stability [10].

Moreover, in some cases diastasis recti plicature, even though is effective, can lead to and excessive tension and therefore increased postoperative pain. In these cases, in our opinion, is necessary to reduce the rectus abdominis suture tension by dividing the external oblique muscle fascia close to the semilunar line and hence medializing the rectus abdominis muscle (*component separation*).

In 1990, Ramirez et al. described the "component separation" technique for the reconstruction of ventral hernias without the use of prosthetic material. Using this technique, up to 10 cm of unilateral recti advancement can be achieved.

On the other hand, it is well known that when an extensive dissection is needed to reach a "component separation", several complications are described (such as hematomas, wound infections, seromas, skin flaps necrosis, etc.). However, many studies report that an optimal compliance of the abdominal wall can be obtained by minimally invasive component separation. It provides up to 86% myofascial advancement compared with an open release [11]. Giurgius et al. compared the conventional component separation technique versus the mini invasive approach for ventral hernias. They concluded that the last one has advantages over the open technique due to a reduction in wound complications. The reduced incidence of seromas seen in the mini invasive approach is likely attributable to the ability to perform the procedure without the creation of undermining skin flaps.

The videoscopic component separation preserves the rectus abdominis myocutaneous perforators supplying the overlying skin and the connection between the subcutaneous fat and anterior rectus sheath, thereby reducing subcutaneous dead space and potentially improving overlying skin flap vascularity. In our opinion, this technique is not only useful for ventral hernia repairs, but also for abdominis diastasis recti surgery. The use of a reinforcing mesh aims to reduce the rate of recurrence.

4. Our experience and conclusion

A total of 42 patients underwent endoscopic surgery between March/2014 and Feb/2017 at British Hospital of Buenos Aires. Most of the patients (76%) were women with a mean age of 39 years and all of them (32) had a history of pregnancy. In 93% (39) of the cases, the diastasis was supra and infraumbilical and its average size was 5.5 cm (range 4–7 cm). About 100% of the patients had at least one associated abdominal wall defect, with the following distributions: 23 umbilical hernias, 18 epigastric hernias, 9 umbilical incisional hernias, and 1 subcostal incisional hernia. We had no intraoperative complications. The mean surgical time was 80 min (55–105 min). Polypropylene meshes were used in 38 patients (91%). Pain intensity at 12 h and at 7 postoperative days was evaluated by analogous visual scale (VAS) and was 4.1 points on average (range 1–6 pts.). The average degree of satisfaction with the cosmetic result was 9.5 with a range of 8–10. All the patients reported being very satisfied with the aesthetic and functional result and the procedure met their preoperative expectations.

Between the 8–10° postoperatory months, the abdominal wall was assessed by ultrasound in 39 patients (93%). After a follow-up of 7–35 months (mean, 10 months), we had no recurrences.

In conclusion, in patients without excess skin or subcutaneous cellular tissue, endoscopic approach to diastasis recti associated with midline hernias is a feasible and reproducible method. It has esthetic advantages, allowing simultaneous correction of all existent pathologies, with minimal complications. Diastasis recti measuring more than 6 cm may benefit with an additional videoscopic component separation technique and/or by using prosthetic mesh.

Laparoscopic approach is also another option for its repair. In this mini-invasive technique, using videoscopic component separation to decrease the tension of the suture between both rectus abdominis is the key to a proper reconstruction.

Author details

Pablo José Medina, Guido Luis Busnelli and Walter Sebastián Nardi*

*Address all correspondence to: nardi.ws@gmail.com

British Hospital of Buenos Aires, Buenos Aires, Argentina

References

[1] Carreirao S, Correa WE, Dias LC, Pitanguy I. Treatment of abdominal wall eventrations associated with abdominoplasty techniques. Aesthetic Plastic Surgery. 1984;8(3):173-179

[2] Ramirez OM. Abdominoplasty and abdominal wall rehabilitation: Comprehensive approach. Plastic and Reconstructive Surgery. 2000;105(1):425-435

[3] Beer GM, Schuster A, Seifert B, Manestar M, Mihic-Probst DA, Weber SA. The normal width of the linea alba in nulliparous women. Clinical Anatomy. 2009;22:706-711

[4] Bellido Luque J, Bellido Luque A, Valdivia J, Suarez Gráu JM, Gomez Menchero J, et al. Totally endoscopic surgery on diastasis recti associated with midline hernias. The advantages of a minimally invasive approach. Prospective cohort study. Hernia. 2015;19(3):493-501

[5] Nahas FX, Ferreira LM, Augusto SM. Ghelfond. Long-term follow-up of correction of rectus diastasis. Plastic and Reconstructive Surgery. 2015;115(6):1736-1741

[6] Mendes Dde A, Nahas FX, Veiga DF. Ultrasonography for measuring rectus abdominis muscles diastasis. Acta Cirúrgica Brasileira. 2007;22:182-186

[7] Yousif NJ, Lifchez SD, Nguyen HH. Transverse rectus sheath plication in abdomino-plasty. Plastic and Reconstructive Surgery. 2004;114:778

[8] Al-Qattan M. Abdominoplasty in multiparous women with severe musculoaponeurotic laxity. British Journal of Plastic Surgery. 1997;50:450-455

[9] Champault G. Video-laparoscopic surgery of the abdominal wall. A study of 15 cases. Chirurgie. 2004;123(5):474-477

[10] Rosen A. Repair of the midline fascial defect in abdominoplasty with long-acting barbed and smooth absorbable sutures. Aesthetic Surgery Journal. 2011;31(6):668-673

[11] Rosen MJ, Williams C, Jin J, McGee MF, Schomisch S, Marks J, Ponsky J. Laparoscopic versus open-component separation: A comparative analysis in porcine model. American Journal of Surgery. 2007;194(3):385-389

Permissions

All chapters in this book were first published in NHLS&LS, by InTech Open; hereby published with permission under the Creative Commons Attribution License or equivalent. Every chapter published in this book has been scrutinized by our experts. Their significance has been extensively debated. The topics covered herein carry significant findings which will fuel the growth of the discipline. They may even be implemented as practical applications or may be referred to as a beginning point for another development.

The contributors of this book come from diverse backgrounds, making this book a truly international effort. This book will bring forth new frontiers with its revolutionizing research information and detailed analysis of the nascent developments around the world.

We would like to thank all the contributing authors for lending their expertise to make the book truly unique. They have played a crucial role in the development of this book. Without their invaluable contributions this book wouldn't have been possible. They have made vital efforts to compile up to date information on the varied aspects of this subject to make this book a valuable addition to the collection of many professionals and students.

This book was conceptualized with the vision of imparting up-to-date information and advanced data in this field. To ensure the same, a matchless editorial board was set up. Every individual on the board went through rigorous rounds of assessment to prove their worth. After which they invested a large part of their time researching and compiling the most relevant data for our readers.

The editorial board has been involved in producing this book since its inception. They have spent rigorous hours researching and exploring the diverse topics which have resulted in the successful publishing of this book. They have passed on their knowledge of decades through this book. To expedite this challenging task, the publisher supported the team at every step. A small team of assistant editors was also appointed to further simplify the editing procedure and attain best results for the readers.

Apart from the editorial board, the designing team has also invested a significant amount of their time in understanding the subject and creating the most relevant covers. They scrutinized every image to scout for the most suitable representation of the subject and create an appropriate cover for the book.

The publishing team has been an ardent support to the editorial, designing and production team. Their endless efforts to recruit the best for this project, has resulted in the accomplishment of this book. They are a veteran in the field of academics and their pool of knowledge is as vast as their experience in printing. Their expertise and guidance has proved useful at every step. Their uncompromising quality standards have made this book an exceptional effort. Their encouragement from time to time has been an inspiration for everyone.

The publisher and the editorial board hope that this book will prove to be a valuable piece of knowledge for researchers, students, practitioners and scholars across the globe.

List of Contributors

Francisco M. Sánchez-Margallo
Jesús Usón Minimally Invasive Surgery Centre, Cáceres, Spain

Juan A. Sánchez-Margallo
Department of Computer Systems and Telematics Engineering, University of Extremadura, Badajoz, Spain

Talha Sarigoz
Department of General Surgery, Sason State Hospital, Batman, Turkey

Inanc Samil Sarici
Department of General Surgery, Kanuni Sultan Suleyman Training and Research Hospital, Istanbul, Turkey

Ozgul Duzgun
Division of Surgical Oncology, Department of General Surgery, Umraniye Training and Research Hospital, Istanbul, Turkey

Mustafa Uygar Kalayci
Department of General Surgery, Kanuni Sultan Suleyman Training and Research Hospital, Istanbul, Turkey

Stefan H. E. M. Clermonts and David D. E. Zimmerman
Department of Surgery, Elisabeth-TweeSteden Hospital, Tilburg, The Netherlands

Laurents P. S. Stassen
Department of Surgery, Maastricht University Medical Center, Maastricht, The Netherlands

Paolo Ialongo and Giuseppe Carbotta
General Surgery Unit, Department of Emergency and Organ Transplantation, School of Medicine, "Aldo Moro", University of Bari, Bari, Italy

Antonio Prestera
General Surgery Unit, Department of Emergency and Organ Transplantation, School of Medicine, "Aldo Moro", University of Bari, Bari, Italy
Surgery Unit, Hospital of Gallipoli, Lecce, Italy

Juan A. Sánchez-Margallo
Department of Medical Technology, SINTEF, Trondheim, Norway
Department of Computer Systems and Telematics Engineering, University of Extremadura, Badajoz, Spain

Thomas Langø and Erlend F. Hofstad
Department of Computer Systems and Telematics Engineering, University of Extremadura, Badajoz, Spain
Norwegian National Advisory Unit on Ultrasound and Image-Guided Therapy, St. Olavs Hospital, Trondheim University Hospital, Trondheim, Norway

Ronald Mårvik
Norwegian National Advisory Unit on Ultrasound and Image-Guided Therapy, St. Olavs Hospital, Trondheim University Hospital, Trondheim, Norway
Department of Gastrointestinal Surgery, St. Olavs Hospital, Trondheim University Hospital, Trondheim, Norway

Francisco M. Sánchez-Margallo
Jesús Usón Minimally Invasive Surgery Centre, Cáceres, Spain

Nidhi Sharma and Vanusha Selvin
Saveetha Medical College, Saveetha University, Chennai, India

Chih Kun Huang, Prasad M. Bhukebag and Khan Wei Chan
Body Science and Metabolic Disorders International (B.M.I.) Medical Center, China Medical University Hospital, Taichung City, Taiwan

Sir Emmanuel S. Astudillo
Center for Diabetes, Nutrition & Weight Management, The Medical City Clark, Pampanga, Philippines

Adrian Kohut and Leah Goldberg
Department of Obstetrics, Gynecology, and Reproductive Sciences, Rutgers Robert Wood Johnson Medical School, Robert Wood Johnson University Hospital, New Brunswick, NJ, United States

Alexandre Buckley De Meritens
Department of Obstetrics, Gynecology, and Reproductive Sciences, Rutgers Robert Wood Johnson Medical School, Robert Wood Johnson University Hospital, New Brunswick, NJ, United States
Division of Gynecologic Oncology, Rutgers Cancer Institute of New Jersey, Robert Wood Johnson University Hospital, New Brunswick, NJ, United States

Arshad M. Malik
College of Medicine, Qassim University, Saudi Arabia

Minako Koizumi, Kei Inaba, Yu Takahashi, Natsuki Nagashima, Hiroshi Ki, Nao Itaoka, Chiharu Ueshima, Maki Nakata and Yoko Hasumi
Department of Obstetrics and Gynecology, Mitsui Memorial Hospital, Tokyo, Japan

Masakazu Sato
Department of Obstetrics and Gynecology, Mitsui Memorial Hospital, Tokyo, Japan
Department of Obstetrics and Gynecology, Graduate School of Medicine, The University of Tokyo, Tokyo, Japan

Pablo José Medina, Guido Luis Busnelli and Walter Sebastián Nardi
British Hospital of Buenos Aires, Buenos Aires, Argentina

Index

www.ingramcontent.com/pod-product-compliance
Lightning Source LLC
Chambersburg PA
CBHW050452200326
41458CB00014B/5150